natural glow

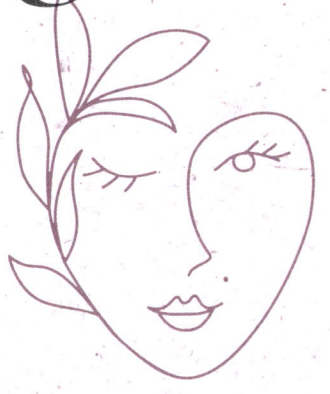

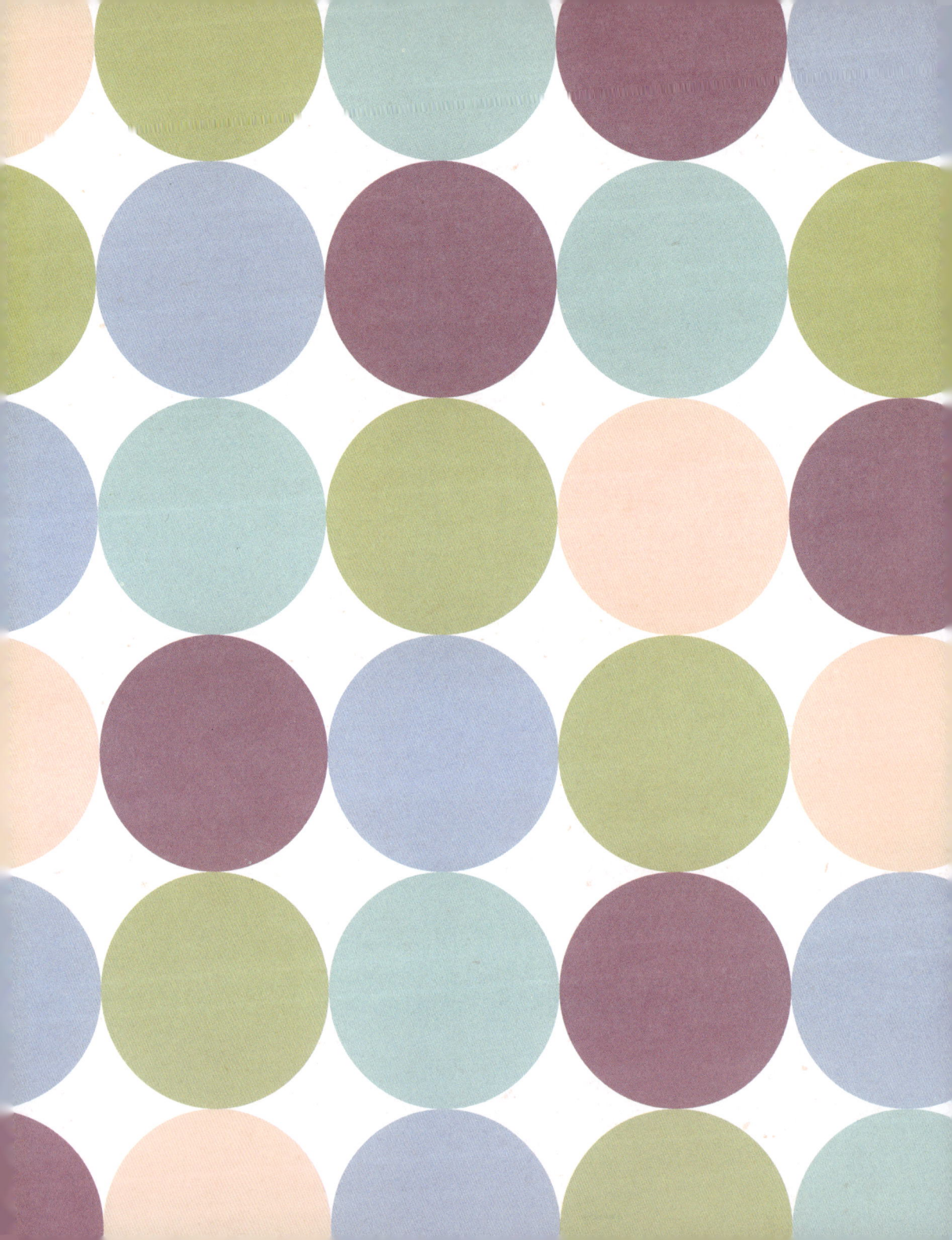

natural glow

FACIAL YOGA, REFLEXOLOGY, OILS, AND MORE FOR RADIANT SKIN

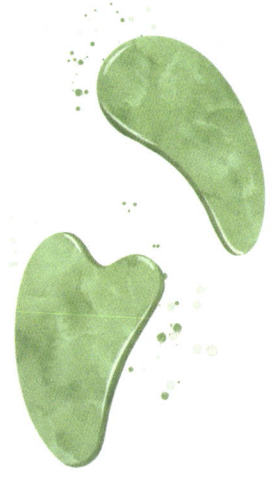

Glenda Taylor

CICO BOOKS

This book is dedicated to my family.

Published in 2025 by CICO Books
An imprint of Ryland Peters & Small Ltd
20–21 Jockey's Fields   1452 Davis Bugg Road
London WC1R 4BW   Warrenton, NC 27589
www.rylandpeters.com
Email: euregulations@rylandpeters.com

10 9 8 7 6 5 4 3 2 1

Text © Glenda Taylor 2025
Design and illustration © CICO Books 2025
For photography credits, see page 128.

The author's moral rights have been asserted.
All rights reserved. No part of this publication
may be reproduced, stored in a retrieval system, or
transmitted in any form or by any means, electronic,
mechanical, photocopying, or otherwise, without
the prior permission of the publisher.

A CIP record for this book is available from the
British Library.
US Library of Congress CIP data has been applied for.

ISBN: 978-1-80065-468-6

Printed in China

Designer: Geoff Borin
Illustrator: Camila Gray

Senior designer: Emily Breen
Art director: Sally Powell
Creative director: Leslie Harrington
Production manager: Gordana Simakovic
Head of production: Patricia Harrington
Publishing manager: Carmel Edmonds

The authorised representative in the EEA is
Authorised Rep Compliance Ltd.,
Ground Floor. 71 Lower Baggot Street,
Dublin, D01 P593, Ireland
www.arccompliance.com

Safety note

Neither the author nor the publisher can be held
responsible for any claim arising out of the general
information and practices provided in this book.
Please note that while the use of particular practices
refer to healing benefits, they are not intended to
replace diagnosis of illness or ailments, or healing or
medicine. Always consult your doctor or other health
professional in the case of illness. If you are pregnant,
have a medical condition, or are on medication, seek
professional advice before trying the practices
provided in this book.

contents

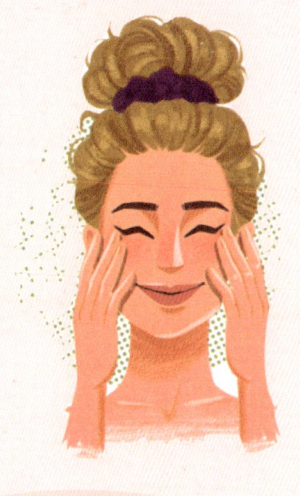

introduction 6

CHAPTER 1: **facial yoga** 8

CHAPTER 2: **facial reflexology** 34

CHAPTER 3: **gua sha and cryotherapy** 56

CHAPTER 4: **recipes for super skin** 72

CHAPTER 5: **natural wellness** 100

resources 125
index 126
acknowledgments 128
photography credits 128

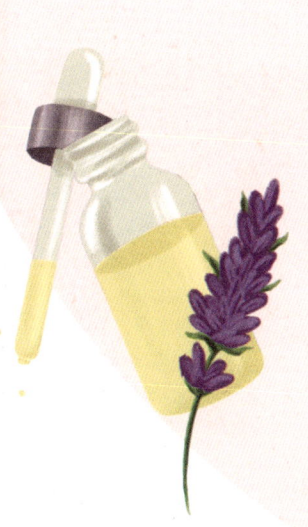

introduction

When I trained to be an aromatherapist more than 30 years ago, I couldn't wait to be older, so that I would be taken seriously. When I told people my plans, I felt that they thought I was jumping on a faddy bandwagon. I am a happy, smiley person, and that sometimes gets mistaken for fluffy! Now, at last, I feel that people believe me when I tell them what an essential oil does or why prevention is always better than cure.

Over the years, I have added other holistic practices to my aromatherapy knowledge base through continuous professional training. Every day is a school day, and you can learn something from everyone. You will see the importance of this reflected in the reflexology and gua sha practices which draw on Traditional Chinese Medicine (see Chapters 2 and 3).

Facial yoga was something of a personal lightbulb moment. When my husband needed speech therapy after a serious illness, we started to add facial yoga exercises to his daily routine, and they worked wonders—so for me there is no doubt about how effective facial yoga can be to make a difference to muscles in the face. It's a natural progression from natural skincare products and massage treatments, so I threw myself into it and have never looked back. Chapter 1 offers a range of exercises which, with time and regular practice, will allow your face to shine.

Natural skincare is something I have always been passionate about. I believe that if you are not comfortable with ingesting your skincare, you shouldn't use it on your face or body. An average of 64 percent of what you put on your skin is absorbed into your body. When you apply a facial skincare product, apart from being absorbed by the skin, quite a lot of the product enters your body through your mouth, inhalation, and even your eyes. I can safely say that there is not one store-bought facial cream, lotion, cleanser, or toner that I would personally be happy to ingest even accidentally! In Chapter 4 you'll learn about how you don't need these artificial products, and how you can embrace all the benefits of natural plant oils.

So, what is a "natural glow"? It is something about a person that literally shines from their very soul—the light that reflects in someone's eyes when they smile or love someone or something deeply. It is something that cannot come out of a bottle. Even with my beloved essential oils, they will only work when care, thought, attention, and intention go into their use. As I often say to my clients, "They won't work if you don't use them!"

Beauty shines from within. You will read in this book how important it is to care for yourself holistically. Holistic means "whole," and that is the central message of this book. Take care of your whole body—which includes your mind—you will be rewarded with a natural glow.

While you may not learn or even embrace everything I have written, I sincerely hope that certain parts will resonate with you and that you will carry them with you through your life. You may even be inspired to expand and improve on them.

Thank you for reading,

Glenda

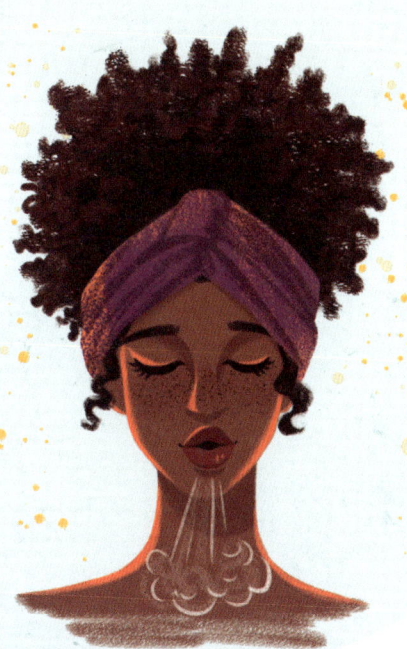

introduction 7

CHAPTER 1

facial yoga

In this chapter you will learn the basics of facial yoga and how to incorporate it into your daily skincare routine. The effectiveness of this well-being habit will literally reflect in your bathroom mirror.

what is facial yoga?

So much more than a natural beauty treatment or regime, facial yoga is a form of well-being that has been around for thousands of years with its roots in ancient India.

Nowadays, facial yoga is prolific across all social marketing platforms with personalized routines, courses, daily exercises, and more. Magazines feature articles about the benefits of facial yoga and celebrities endorse it regularly. At the same time, Botox and other injectables are also growing in popularity, but chemical intervention is not without risk, and for those who prefer a natural glow, face yoga is a brilliant alternative.

The word "yoga" comes from the Sanskrit word *yuj* which means "union," and this refers, loosely speaking, to the union of body, mind, soul, and spirit. If we can master this union, we are sure to look and feel on top of the world.

Facial yoga is an extension of full body yoga and if you have practiced yoga already, you will almost certainly have come across some of the exercises you will find in this book (see Kiss the Sky on page 23 and Eye Freshener on page 19). However, to perform facial yoga, you do not need to change your clothes, lay out your mat, or do anything other than carry out your chosen exercises while looking in the mirror each morning and/or night, and it only takes a few minutes. Here lies one of the many beauties of facial yoga: its simplicity and ease.

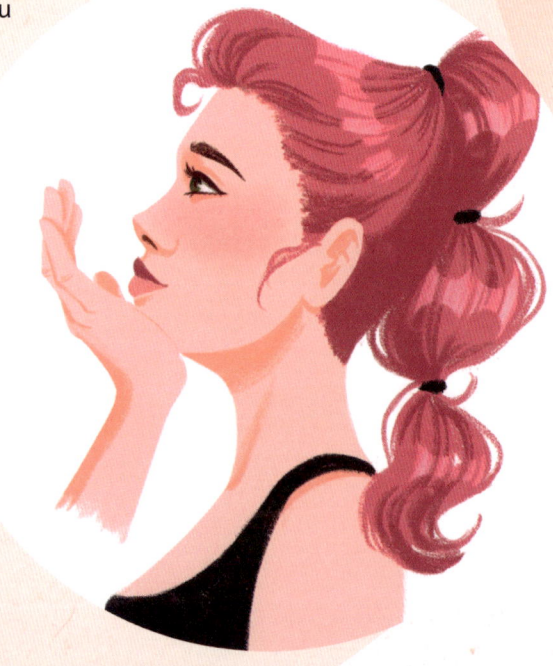

10 facial yoga

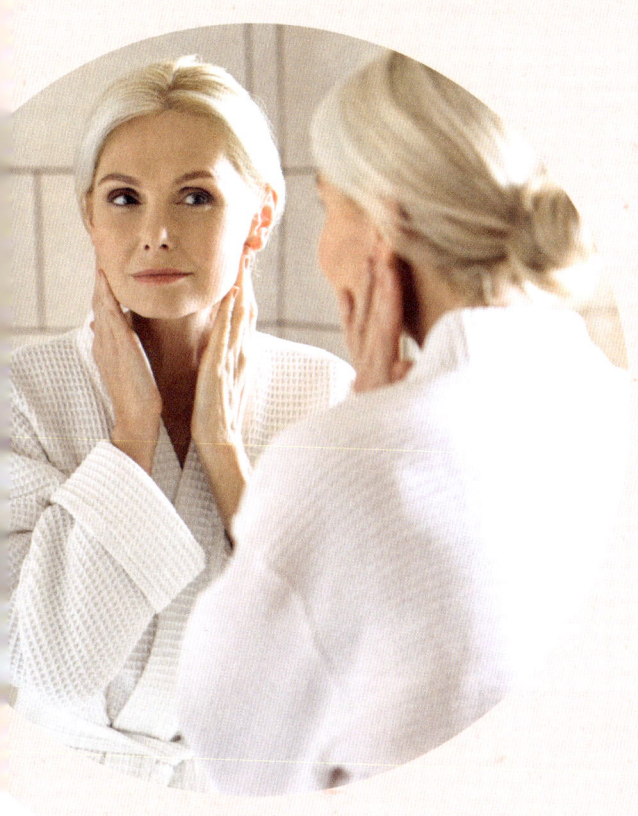

benefits of facial yoga

- Glowing complexion
- Facial definition
- Sense of calm and control
- Better elocution
- Clear head
- Better posture
- Smoother skin
- Better facial symmetry
- Reduced puffiness
- Peachy cheeks and lips
- Longer, smoother neck
- Improved mood

how can facial yoga help?

There are myriad good reasons to make facial yoga part of your lifestyle, and they will almost certainly be different for everyone.

You may want to make minor cosmetic improvements, such as reducing fine lines, asymmetry of the face, or puffiness. However, facial yoga can also be helpful for speech problems, whether from an accident, a medical procedure, or an impediment. Even a habit or twitch, like biting the inside of your mouth or sniffing, can be unlearned and replaced with a good facial yoga routine.

a change of expression

A change of expression can mean a change of direction. If you've been feeling stuck in a rut, you might find that a change of expression will give you a different outlook.

Like it or not, people often unwittingly judge us by our expression. If we scowl or frown all the time, we will be judged as moody, even by people who have never met us before. The sad thing is that we might not even be feeling that way. We may have become so used to making this expression, maybe learned from our parents or a teacher when we were very young, that the muscles in our forehead have "set" in that position. To correct this, we simply need to reset our muscles by teaching them an alternative position—which can only be done through repetition.

Once you have ironed out any expressions that you feel are not serving you well, you can replace them with more positive ones, which includes smiling more. There have been many studies on the benefits of smiling, and training yourself to smile more often is definitely a form of facial yoga.

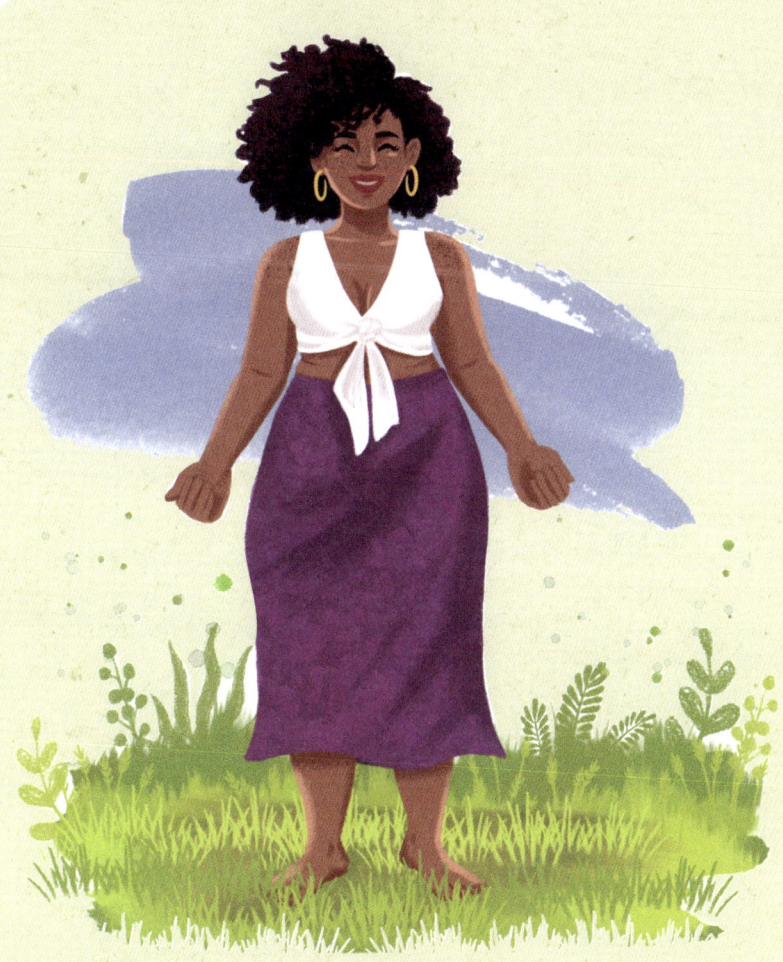

You will notice that some of the exercises listed in this book rely on a smile. A simple smile not only requires the use of many facial and even neck muscles, but also releases endorphins, dopamine, and serotonin, which can all improve your mood dramatically, even when you are "fake smiling." Indeed, it is very difficult to hold on to sad or angry thoughts while smiling. Try it!

how can facial yoga help?

how does facial yoga work?

Your face has approximately 43 muscles and your neck has more than 20. That's a lot of muscles for a small area! Giving some of these muscles a workout will plump them up and give your skin a better support structure.

We don't question that going to the gym, running, cycling, swimming, or any other physical activity will improve our fitness as well as our overall look. This is because we know that by strengthening and working our muscles, we will pump blood into them, sculpt them, and in turn burn off excess fat. Simple daily activity will do this to a certain extent, including walking, getting up and down from a chair, bending down, and picking up things (or children). However, targeted exercises will sculpt and tone.

Similarly, we eat, speak, frown, and smile, and these activities work well enough to keep our faces functioning, but if we want our look to "glow," like our well-exercised bodies, we need to exercise our face and neck muscles.

The great news is that it doesn't matter what age you are. Some of the exercises might be a little tiring to begin with, but you will build up muscle and stamina quickly and this will be a good sign that you are progressing.

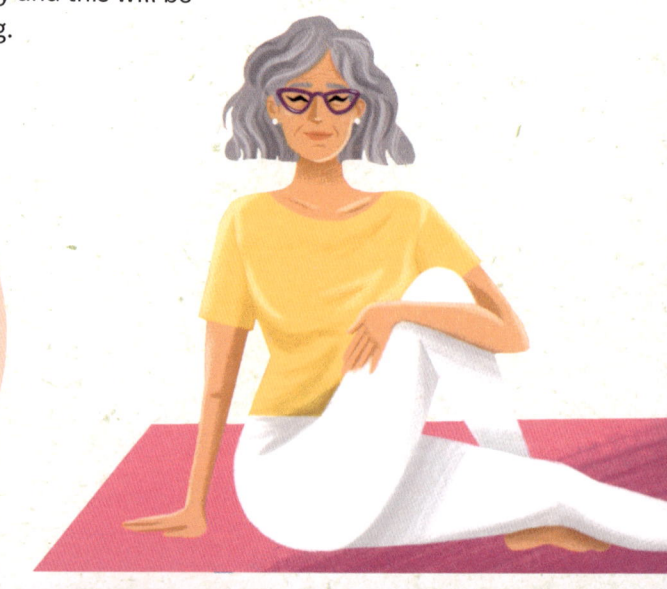

CAUTION

Never strain while doing facial yoga and never hold poses for too long. You don't need to feel a "burn." The aim is to gently build up strength and stamina.

developing a habit

To achieve a natural glow, I encourage you to learn the two-minute routine on pages 18–21 and use it daily. When you're comfortable with it, you can add to it and make it longer and more targeted to specific areas of your face or neck using the exercises on pages 22–29 if you wish. You could also take a facial yoga class or add facial yoga exercises to your regular yoga practice, if you have one, but to really see results in your face and neck you need to practice your chosen exercises regularly. It takes 30 days to make a habit stick, so challenge yourself to do this short routine each morning for at least a month and bask in the results.

INSTANT RELAXATION

When you are feeling tense, try placing the heel of one hand at the top of your nose, with your palm over your forehead and your fingers toward the crown of your head. Relax your forehead, close your eyes, and take a few deep breaths. This teaches you not to send tension and lines directly to your forehead and is a great relaxation tool.

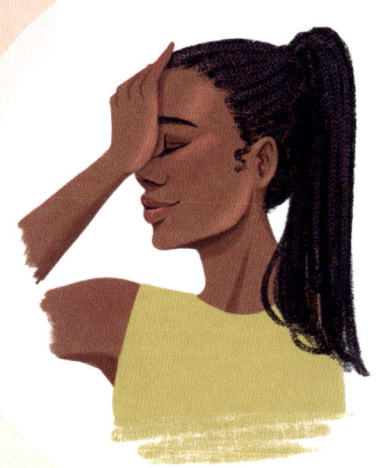

how does facial yoga work?

getting prepared

Just as you need to warm up your body before you begin a traditional yoga sequence, so too should you prepare yourself for facial yoga to fully reap the benefits.

posture and breath

To perform facial yoga exercises efficiently, you need to think about your posture. Standing or sitting up straight, with your shoulders down and your neck long, gives your lungs "room" to fill with air. Breathing well improves circulation, which in turn enhances your complexion.

My yoga teacher nearly always begins her class by saying, "Bring your attention to your breath." It is the same with facial yoga: begin with a few deep, conscious breaths. Think about lengthening your spine while your breaths become longer and more rhythmic. If you wish, continue the breathwork while you are doing the exercises. Performing the exercises rhythmically will help them become second nature over time and the rhythm will make it easier for you to focus.

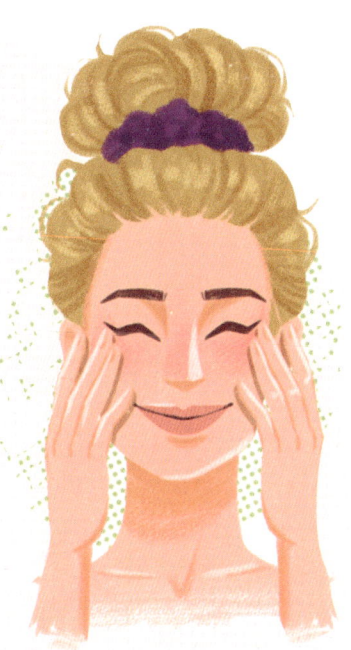

preparing the skin

It is not at all necessary to use oils for facial yoga. A simple face and neck cleanse, or even starting yoga straight after a shower, will suffice. However, you may like to add them as part of your routine, just as I do—I love the ritual.

I do my face yoga every morning. After my shower, with my hair back in a towel, I spray a natural hydrosol (flower water—see page 92) over my face and neck, and then apply my favorite facial oil (see page 96). I massage the oil all over my face and neck, which allows me to identify any areas which feel slightly achy to the touch and are therefore holding stress or fatigue, so I can give them a little more massage while my skin soaks up the beautiful plant oils.

warming up and cooling down

For a longer, more in-depth home facial yoga session, it's a good idea to warm up and cool down. A technique that you might enjoy using is what I call "raindrop fingers."

Simply tap the fingers of both hands all over your face and neck like raindrops for 1–2 minutes. You only need to do this very lightly for it to be both relaxing and invigorating. You will love the feeling.

getting prepared 17

two-minute morning routine

It is so easy to incorporate facial yoga into your morning routine—and also fun and invigorating! You will quickly build muscle and tone in your face, giving it a younger, fresher, and more dynamic look.

This sequence is long enough to be effective, yet short enough for there to be absolutely no reason not to do it. Habit is the key to success. By performing the routine daily, it will become second nature, so you automatically segue into your morning facial yoga straight after washing or cleansing.

The routine below includes one simple exercise for each part of your face and neck, but if there are particular areas that you feel need more work, you could either repeat the exercises for those from this routine or add a couple more from the exercises on pages 22–23. The exercises can be completed in any order, but it is best to work up or down the face in a methodical way as this helps you to learn the steps more easily.

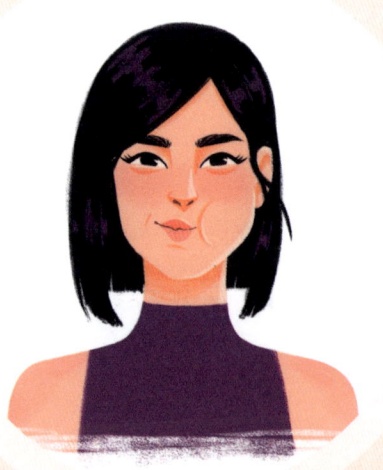

cheek plumper

1 With your mouth closed, fill your left cheek with air and hold for 5 seconds.

2 Open your mouth and push the air out quickly with force.

3 Repeat steps 1–2 with your right cheek. Repeat alternate cheeks four more times.

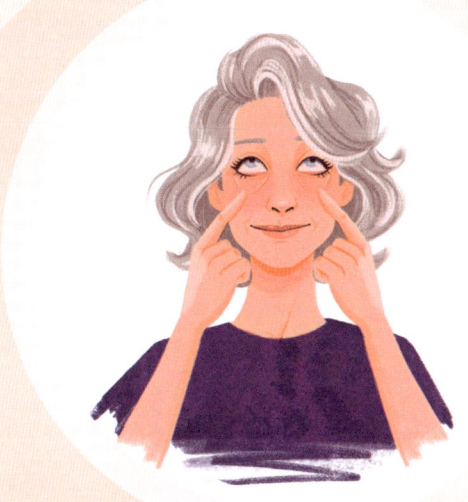

eye freshener

1 Using your index fingers, gently pull your under eye "bags" down while looking up. Hold for 5 seconds.

2 Rest for a couple of seconds, then repeat step 1 twice more.

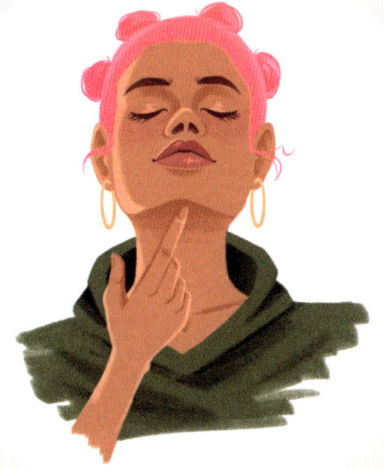

neck beautifier

1 Gently tip your head backward as far as is comfortable for you, being careful not to scrunch the back of your neck.

2 Place your index finger on the tip of your chin and stick your chin out while gently pressing it with your finger. Hold for 5 seconds.

3 Bring your head back to its normal position and rest for a couple of seconds, then repeat steps 1–2 five more times.

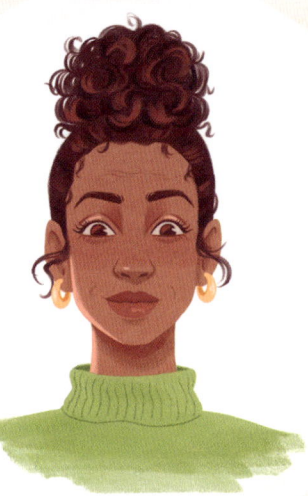

forehead smoother

1 Raise your eyebrows and look upward for 5 seconds, then frown looking downward for 5 seconds. Repeat five times.

2 Rest for a couple of seconds, then repeat step 1 twice more.

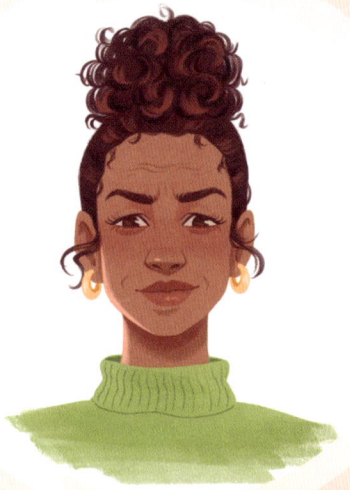

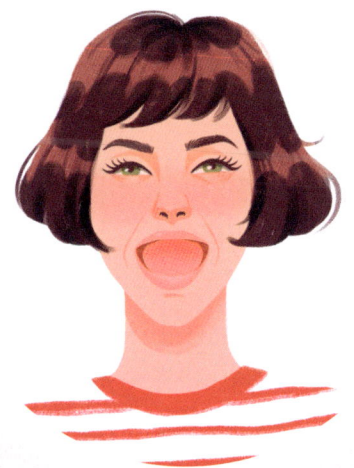

mouth refiner

1 Open your mouth wide and cover your teeth with your lips.

2 Staying in this position, make a smile and then an "O." Repeat five times.

3 Rest for a couple of seconds, then repeat steps 1–2 once more.

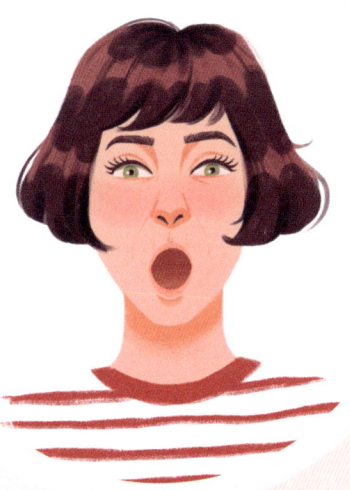

nose conditioner

1 Wrinkle up your nose as if something smells bad. Hold for 5 seconds.

2 Rest for a couple of seconds, then repeat step 1 twice more.

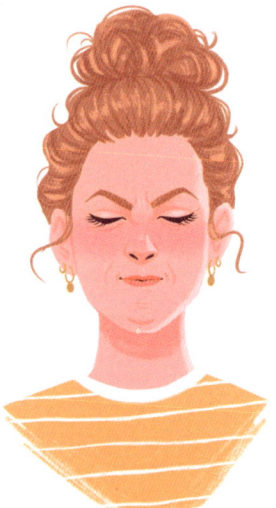

two-minute morning routine 21

for a strong, long neck

When thinking about exercises for the neck, we include the jawline, as most facial yoga exercises will help add definition to the jaw as well as improving the appearance of the neck.

As well as trying the exercises here, you can adjust the appearance of saggy neck skin and double chins by improving your posture. Lowering your shoulders and lifting your chin slightly will give an instant "ballerina" look. When you have developed enough strength to hold this position without thinking, people will soon be asking what you have been doing to look so healthy, toned, and well!

vowel shapes

In this exercise you will feel the muscles in your neck and jaw working. Remember to keep your shoulders down throughout the sequence. For each vowel shape, you can also make the sound while doing it, or stay silent—whichever you prefer.

1 Open your mouth into a big "O" shape, holding for 5 seconds.

2 Now make an "E" shape, followed by a "U" shape, again holding each one for 5 seconds.

3 Repeat the sequence of O, E, U ten times.

supple neck

This sequence combines spine alignment and neck stretches.

1 Making sure you are sitting or standing up straight, with your shoulders down, slide your head forward like a chicken and then slide it right back toward your neck. (The person who taught me this technique likes to call it the funky chicken move!) This aligns your spine.

2 Keeping your head in the same position, turn your head to the right, then look down toward your right shoulder, holding for 10 seconds. When you look down to the side, you should feel a lovely stretch at the back of your neck. Lift your chin back up to a straight position again, then turn back to face the front.

3 Repeat step 1 to realign your spine, then repeat step 2 on the left side.

4 Repeat steps 1–3 three times.

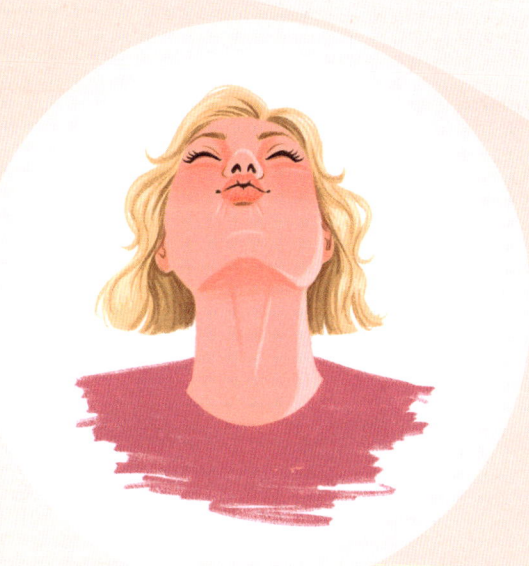

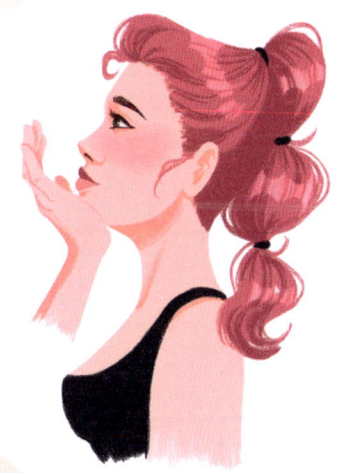

kiss the sky

For this neck stretch, be careful to keep your shoulders down and ensure you are not scrunching the back of your neck.

1 Lift your chin slightly and purse your lips as if you are kissing the sky, then make a big smile, holding each pose for 5 seconds. Really exaggerate each movement.

2 Alternate between kissing and smiling five times.

neck strengthener

If you experience a lot of neck pain or headaches, this exercise may help. You will feel the muscles in the back of your neck working, and this will help support your head.

1 Place the heel of your hand under your chin. Press your chin into your hand while also pushing it up, holding for 10 seconds.

2 Repeat step 1 five times.

3 Rest and roll your shoulders a few times to relax.

4 Repeat step 1 twice more.

for a strong, long neck

for a smooth forehead

There are two types of lines that appear on the forehead: vertical lines, called glabella lines and better known as frown lines, and horizontal lines, which appear over the frontalis muscle of the forehead.

Vertical frown lines appear at the top of the nose, between the eyebrows. When we are young, these lines are dynamic, which means they only appear when we are actually frowning, but as time goes by, the lines can embed themselves and become more permanent. This is also the position of the Third Eye, which is said to focus on intuition and awareness, and it is an extremely relaxing area to massage (see Five-minute Evening Routine, Step 4 on page 49).

Horizonal lines on the forehead develop from repeatedly raising your eyebrows. Some people do this whenever they look up, but it is possible to train yourself to keep your forehead relaxed when moving your eyes, and this can give your forehead a much smoother appearance.

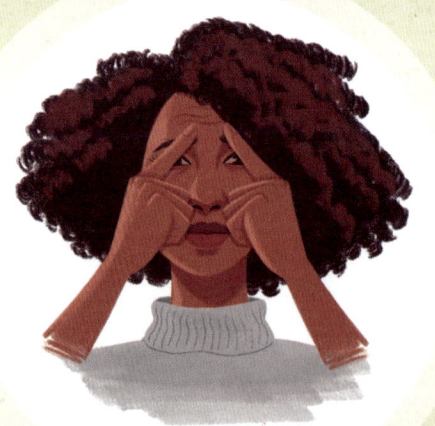

frown-line reducer

The resistance against your fingers in this exercise engages the corrugator muscle between your eyebrows, which helps to smooth your frown lines.

1 Place both your index fingers over your frown lines.

2 Gently move your fingers apart by just a few millimeters, then frown while trying to keep the fingers apart. Hold for 5 seconds.

3 Relax and repeat steps 1–2 five times.

24   facial yoga

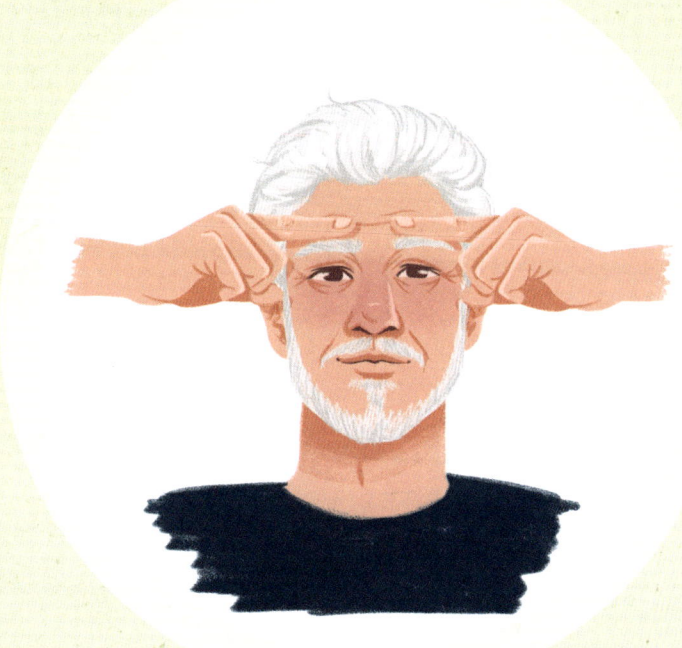

forehead isolation

This exercise can be quite tiring for the eyes, so only do it once or twice if you find it a strain. It will become easier over time.

1 Lower your chin and look down.

2 Now look up while keeping your chin down but without raising your eyebrows or wrinkling your forehead. Keep looking up for 5 seconds.

3 Relax your eyes and lift your chin to a neutral position.

4 Repeat steps 1–3 three times.

horizontal-line reducer

This exercise works in much the same way as the frown-line reducer, but in a different direction, so you are working on the horizontal forehead lines.

1 Place the side of your index fingers just above your eyebrows, then gently press down toward your eyes.

2 Now try to lift your eyebrows while maintaining a gentle downward pressure. Hold for 5 seconds.

3 Relax and repeat steps 1–2 five times.

for a smooth forehead

for peachy cheeks

Laughter lines are the main lines that appear around the cheeks with age. Even though this might be a sign of a happy life, laughter lines can also come from saggy cheeks and jowls.

The good news is that we can plump these areas up a little with exercise and massage. Simply smiling also engages the muscles of the cheeks. You will see that two of the exercises on these pages are based around a smile.

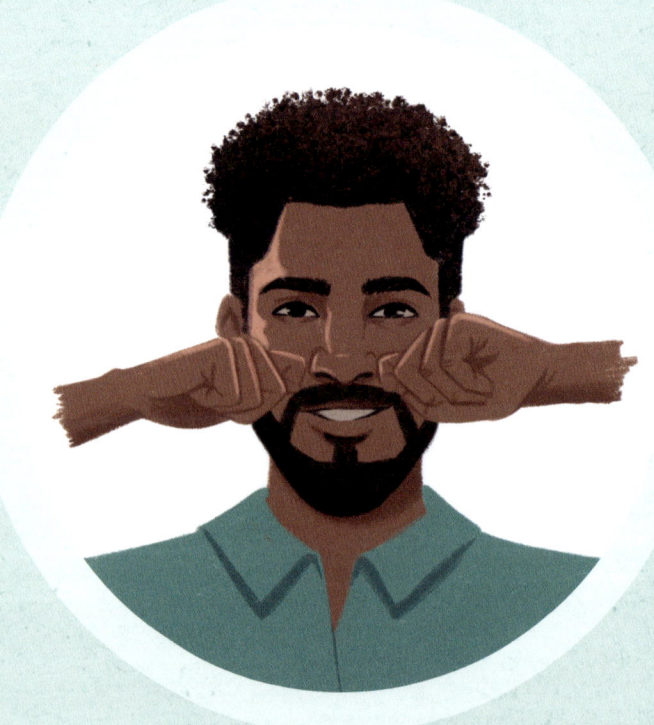

fish hooks

This is a very satisfying exercise. Your "fish hooks" will feel as though they are literally erasing lines.

1 Make a hook with both index fingers. You are now going to use your middle knuckle to stroke the laughter lines. Place the "hooks" at the base of both sides of your nose.

2 Make a big smile and gently trace under your cheeks with your hooked fingers. Relax between each stroke and repeat five times.

fish mouth

Children are really good at doing this exercise. As we get older, we often lose the ability to make a fish mouth.

1 With your mouth closed and teeth slightly apart, suck in your cheeks, being careful not to bite the insides of your cheeks. Try to purse your lips into a fish-like mouth.

2 Open and close your lips three times, then relax.

3 Now repeat steps 1–2 five times.

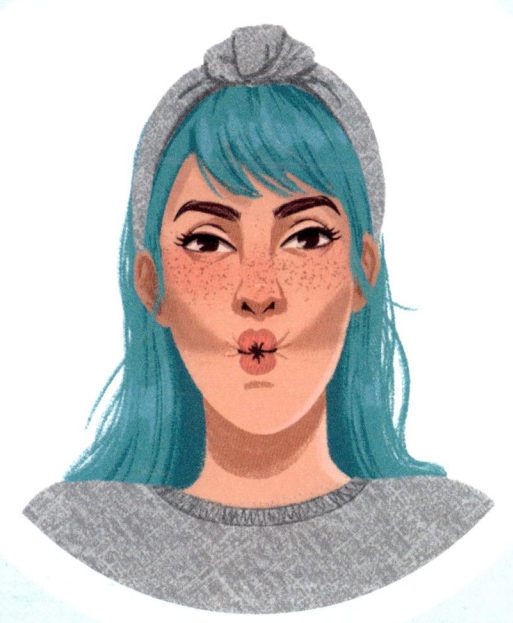

smile, smile, smile

This exercise is so called because you do three degrees of smile.

1 Make a small smile with your mouth closed, holding for 3 seconds.

2 Next, make a slightly bigger smile with your mouth closed, holding for 3 seconds.

3 Make a big smile, showing your teeth, again holding for 3 seconds.

4 Relax, then repeat steps 1–3 five times.

for peachy cheeks

for a happy mouth

Lips are the most popular area to have pumped up with injectables, such as Botox. However, it is possible to improve their appearance with these natural techniques instead.

Full lips are often considered a sign of beauty, but unfortunately, lips can very easily become thin and lined. Toxins found in cigarettes can dehydrate the delicate area around the lips, leaving them saggy and lined. These tiny lines are often called smoke lines and can make a person look prematurely old. Massaging and exercising the area around the lips can increase the production of collagen, which in turn can give the appearance of plumper lips.

kiss kiss: warm-up for the mouth

Start your mouth facial yoga exercises by sending yourself kisses in the mirror, exaggerating your pout with each kiss. Twenty kisses will warm you up nicely!

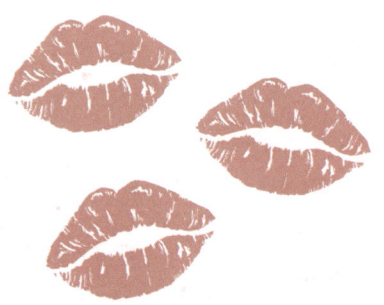

tongue twister

As well as giving your lips a more glowing look, mouth exercises can be very good for improving diction. This exercise strengthens the tongue and helps to reduce fine lines around the lips. Try not to move your chin too much while doing this exercise. By keeping your chin as still as possible, your tongue has to work harder.

1 With your mouth closed, trace the inside of your lips three times with the tip of your tongue, starting at the middle of your top lip and moving your tongue in a clockwise circle via the side of your top lip, your bottom lip, and the other side of your top lip, before returning to top center. Repeat this in a counterclockwise direction. Relax for a moment.

2 Repeat three times in each direction twice more.

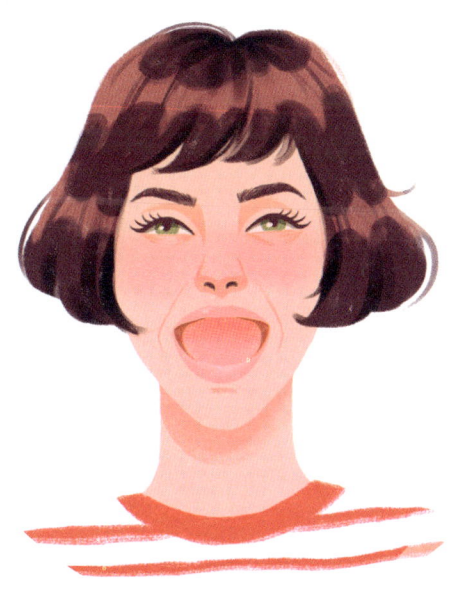

lip line reducer

Work on smoothing those smoke lines with this simple exercise.

1 Cover your teeth with your lips, then open your mouth wide, holding for 5 seconds.

2 Now make a small "ooh" shape for 5 seconds, while still keeping your teeth covered with your lips.

3 Repeat steps 1–2 four times, making five rounds in total.

4 Relax, then repeat the five rounds again.

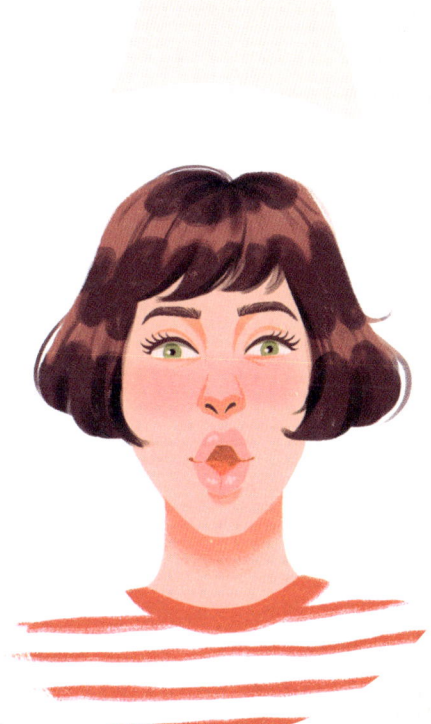

for a happy mouth

for bright eyes

There was a time when eye exercises were taught in schools to improve eyesight and concentration. While doing the exercises below, you will really feel the muscles of your eyes working. They will soon look and feel brighter.

The skin around the eyes is 40 percent thinner than anywhere else on the body, so care needs to be taken whenever you cleanse, massage, or even just touch this area. Since it is so delicate, it has a tendency to sag and wrinkle very easily. Constant poor lifestyle choices will reflect in your eyes. Overdrinking, overeating, and smoking, as well as lack of sleep, are all reflected in the area around your eyes.

crow's feet minimizer

The fine lines that form at the outer corners of your eyes are called lateral canthal lines, but are better known as crow's feet. This exercise is wonderfully simple but effective. It also gives you the opportunity to open your eyes wide while trying to keep your forehead smooth, which is one of the best ways to stop new lines from appearing on the forehead.

1 Simply open your eyes as wide as possible and stare into the distance, holding for 10 seconds. While doing this, check by feeling with your fingers or looking in a mirror that your forehead and the area where crow's feet appear are as smooth as possible. Then relax the eyes.

2 Repeat step 1 five times.

30 facial yoga

around the clock

This exercise can be helpful for dry eyes as it can stimulate them to produce moisture. You might find when you are doing this exercise that your eyes water a little, but this is a good thing. They are simply reacting to the air and movement.

1 Look straight ahead with your eyes wide open and your forehead relaxed.

2 Look to the right, keeping your head still, and hold for 5 seconds.

3 Look down, holding for 5 seconds.

4 Look to the left, holding for 5 seconds.

5 Look up, holding for 5 seconds.

6 Repeat steps 2–5 twice more, then relax.

7 Repeat the whole sequence of steps 2–6 the other way—that is, looking left, down, right, and up.

lid and brow lift

This is another exercise that may make your eyes water a little, but it is also very refreshing for them.

1 Put the side of each index finger under your eyebrows. Gently use your fingers to lift your brows, and counteract this movement by making your brows push down against your fingers. Hold for 5 seconds, then relax.

2 Repeat step 1 four times.

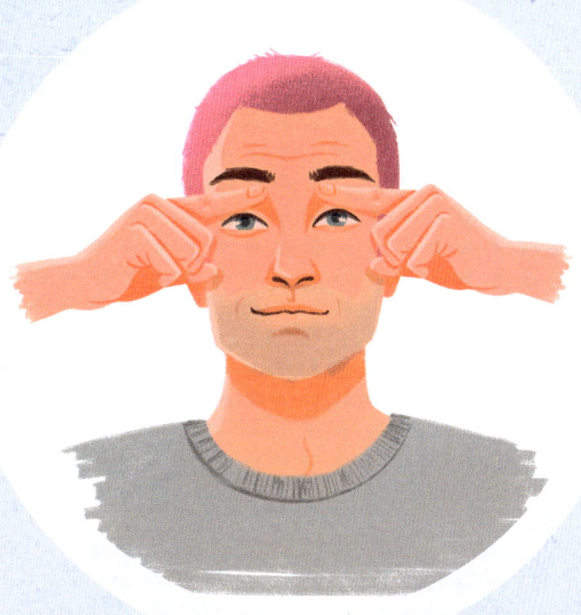

for bright eyes

for a fine nose

As we get older, our nose has a tendency to spread a little. This is because the muscles and cartilage weaken. Exercising the nose can give a more toned appearance. It is not the easiest area to work on, but it is worth persevering and the results can be very pleasing.

nose massage: warm-up for the nose

This massage is not only very relaxing, but it will also stimulate blood circulation in this area ready for exercises. Using the index finger of your dominant hand, make small circular massage movements all over the nose, working all the way down the length of your nose from the bridge to the tip and then covering each side. Work into every little area.

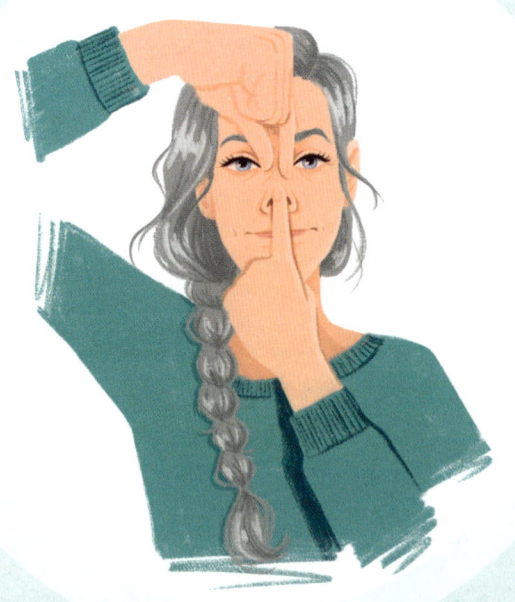

nose flex

This is real workout for your nose and upper lip. Both will feel energized after doing this exercise.

1 Hold the bridge of your nose with the thumb and forefinger of one hand. With the index finger of your other hand, gently push up the tip of your nose. Pull your top lip over your teeth. Hold for 5 seconds, then relax.

2 Repeat step 1 four times.

nose flare

Simply flaring your nostrils—allowing them to widen while breathing—uses the nasalis muscles, which can become lazy and floppy.

1 Flare your nostrils three times during one deep breath in, then flare another three times to one deep breath out, then relax.

2 Repeat step 1 four times.

breath push

This exercise is an extension of the Nose Flare exercise, in which you also apply pressure to the nasalis muscles, just like resistance exercises at the gym.

1 Place your index fingers on the side of each nostril with a little pressure, but making sure to leave room for air to enter and exit.

2 As you breathe in for 4 counts, flare your nostrils against your fingers. Remove your fingers as you breathe out, then relax for a moment.

3 Repeat steps 1–2 five more times.

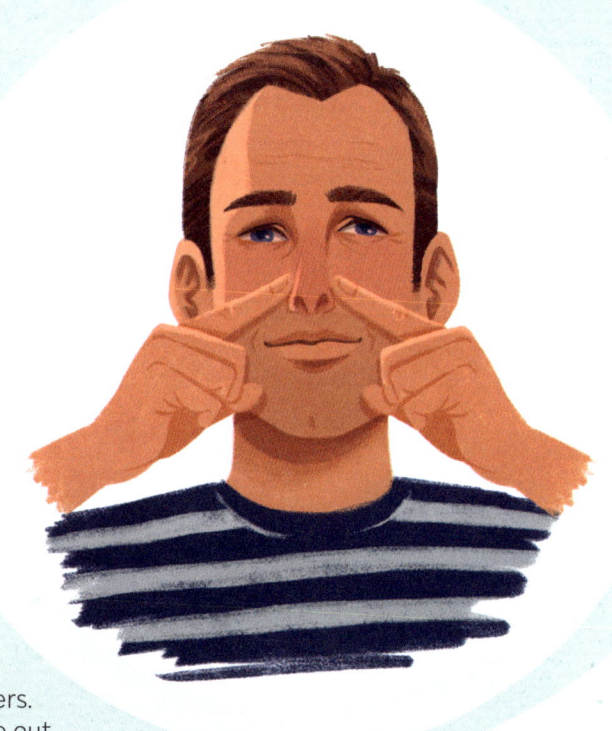

for a fine nose 33

CHAPTER 2

facial reflexology

Even though this book concentrates on achieving a natural glow on your face and neck, this would be impossible without thinking of the body as a whole. Reflexology is a holistic treatment and holistic means whole. A happy, healthy body results in a vibrant, glowing look. Therefore, what could be better than a facial treatment that addresses imbalances in the body? Pure synergy!

what is facial reflexology?

This wonderfully relaxing treatment not only brings a glow to your face and neck, but also has the added advantage of addressing energy blockages throughout the body.

Facial reflexology stems from Traditional Chinese Medicine (TCM). TCM states that chi or qi—that is, energy—runs throughout our bodies through channels called meridians. However, the chi can get blocked, causing ill health both physically and mentally. Certain points or zones are connected to other parts of the body by the meridians. By stimulating these points, energy and blood is sent around the body from the area being stimulated to its corresponding zone.

This concept has been used for more than 6,000 years and it forms the basis of acupuncture, which uses needles to stimulate the relevant points, and reflexology, where massage with the hands or simple tools are used instead. There are different types of reflexology—foot, hand, and ear, as well as facial.

With facial reflexology, by gently stimulating the corresponding reflex points, you can give what ultimately feels like a full body massage simply by working on the face. This concept may be easier to understand when you look at the charts on pages 38–41.

the history of facial reflexology

Nhuan Le Quang, an architect living in South Vietnam in the 1980s, consulted an acupuncture clinic run by Professor Bùi Quốc Châu for his chronic asthma. The clinic offered a kind of facial acupuncture. He found this treatment very successful in easing his asthma symptoms. Wanting to take his health into his own hands, he mirrored the techniques performed with needles at Professor Bùi Quốc Châu's clinic using a simple ballpoint pen to stimulate the reflex points on his face. Nhuan Le Quang moved to Paris to be with his family and continued to study Professor Bùi Quốc Châu's principles but without the use of needles. He developed the facial reflexology treatment and, in doing so, expanded its popularity in the West. Nowadays, facial reflexology is usually done alongside facial massage, facial yoga, and gua sha (see page 56), giving a rounded treatment that can be very effective.

TRY IT YOURSELF

If you are feeling tense, rubbing up and down the nose can "sedate" or relax the spine.

•

For bloating from overeating, a circular massage around the mouth can be helpful. Simply trace the outside of your lips all the way around your mouth with an index or middle finger in a smooth, rhythmic movement. You might want to open your mouth a little when you do this. Repeat ten times.

•

To feel relaxed in moments, gently massage the two small areas on the forehead as shown on the right.

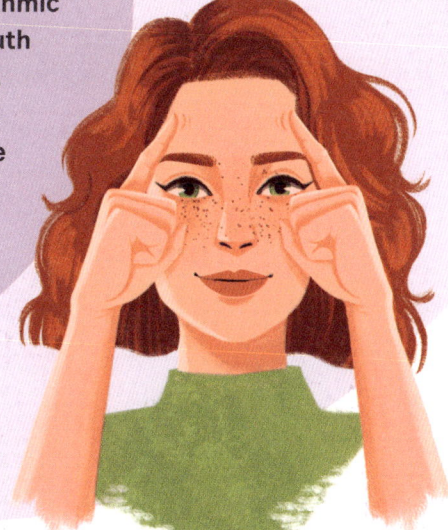

what is facial reflexology?

facial reflexology charts

As explained on the previous pages, there are reflex points on the face which connect to different parts of the body. Here, we explore what those connections are.

There are many different charts for facial reflexology. All are based on the principle found in the *I Ching*, an ancient book of Chinese wisdom, which states that "what resembles, assembles"—meaning that a buildup of stagnant energy and blockages assemble in areas that mirror the "look" of the body.

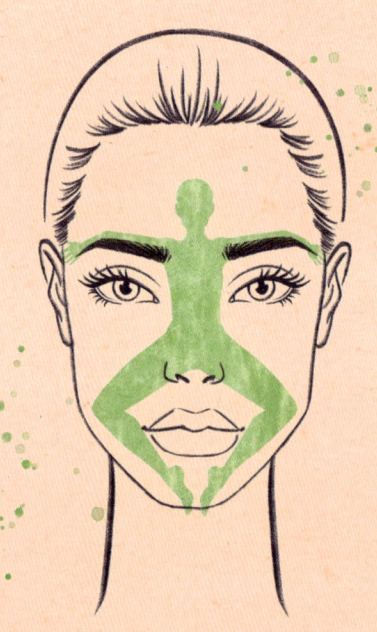

In this chart, the head zone is shown on the forehead with the spine running down the nose, legs either side of the mouth, and arms across the forehead.

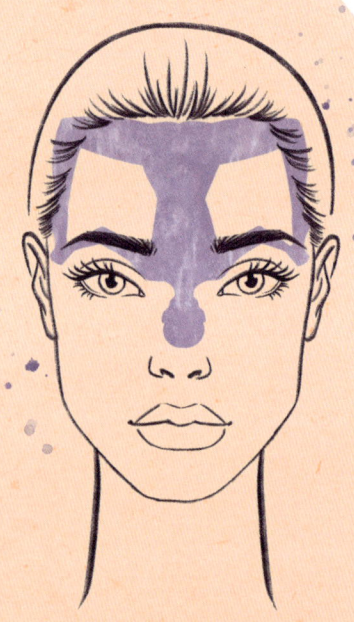

In contrast, this chart shows almost the complete opposite, with the neck vertebrae between the eyes, and the coccyx (base of the spine) at the very top of the forehead. Here, the arms are still running across the eyebrows.

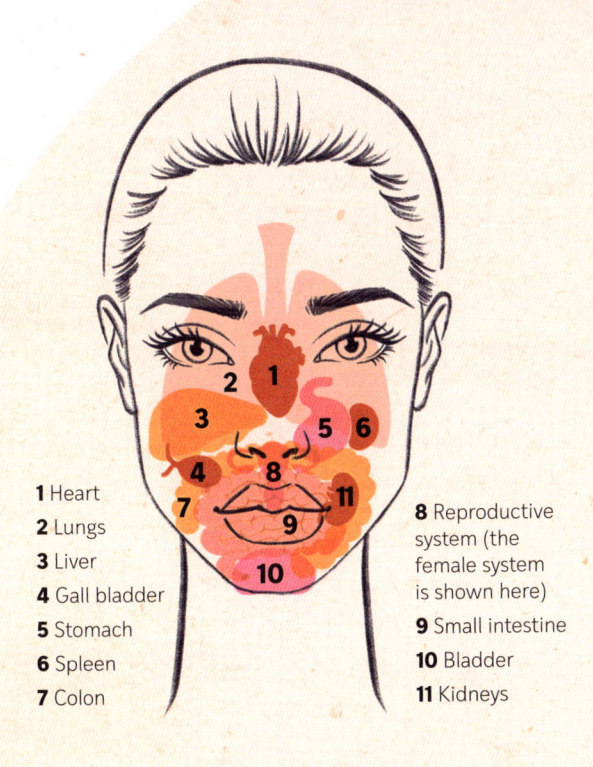

1 Heart
2 Lungs
3 Liver
4 Gall bladder
5 Stomach
6 Spleen
7 Colon
8 Reproductive system (the female system is shown here)
9 Small intestine
10 Bladder
11 Kidneys

This version links areas of the face to organs of the body.

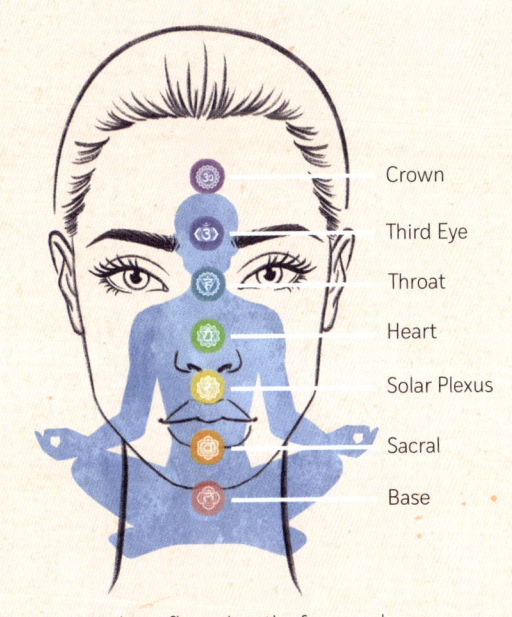

- Crown
- Third Eye
- Throat
- Heart
- Solar Plexus
- Sacral
- Base

Chakras are also reflected on the face, as shown here. Chakras are energy points on the body, which again are linked by meridians. Like reflex points, there are many chakras on the body, but there are seven major ones: Crown, Third Eye, Throat, Heart, Solar Plexus, Sacral, and Base. Find out more about the chakras on pages 106–107.

reflexology in practice

These charts may seem very confusing, and it can take a long time to become familiar with them. However, for a natural glow, you only need to know the principles to achieve great results. On the following pages, we will work with 11 facial reflex points which draw from all the charts here and are the ones most used in treatments. They are much simpler to understand and remember.

facial reflexology charts

eleven facial reflex zones

As an introduction to facial reflexology, we are using just 11 reflex points or zones of the face that cover some organs and joints, plus relaxation and chakra points for a holistic treatment that can be learned and used by anyone.

The chart opposite shows where the 11 reflex zones are located on the face. It may be difficult to remember them all as a beginner. Find the ones that are most useful to you and expand your knowledge over time. You will see that there is more than one point for every area. This is because meridians loop around the body like a spaghetti junction and reflex points will show up in several areas. Learn the ones that are most obvious to you.

A fun experiment to try is to press around your face for sensitive areas and then look up what those areas signify on your charts. It is fascinating that almost without exception they will mirror imbalances in the body that you were already aware of.

You might wonder why these reflex zone numbers are so random. As described earlier, there are many charts, meridians, and chakras. I have chosen the ones that I thought would work best for this routine. I could have numbered them 1 to 11, but then when you come to learn from other sources, the numbers would be wrong and wouldn't match up, so here I have given you the classic building blocks from which to expand your knowledge.

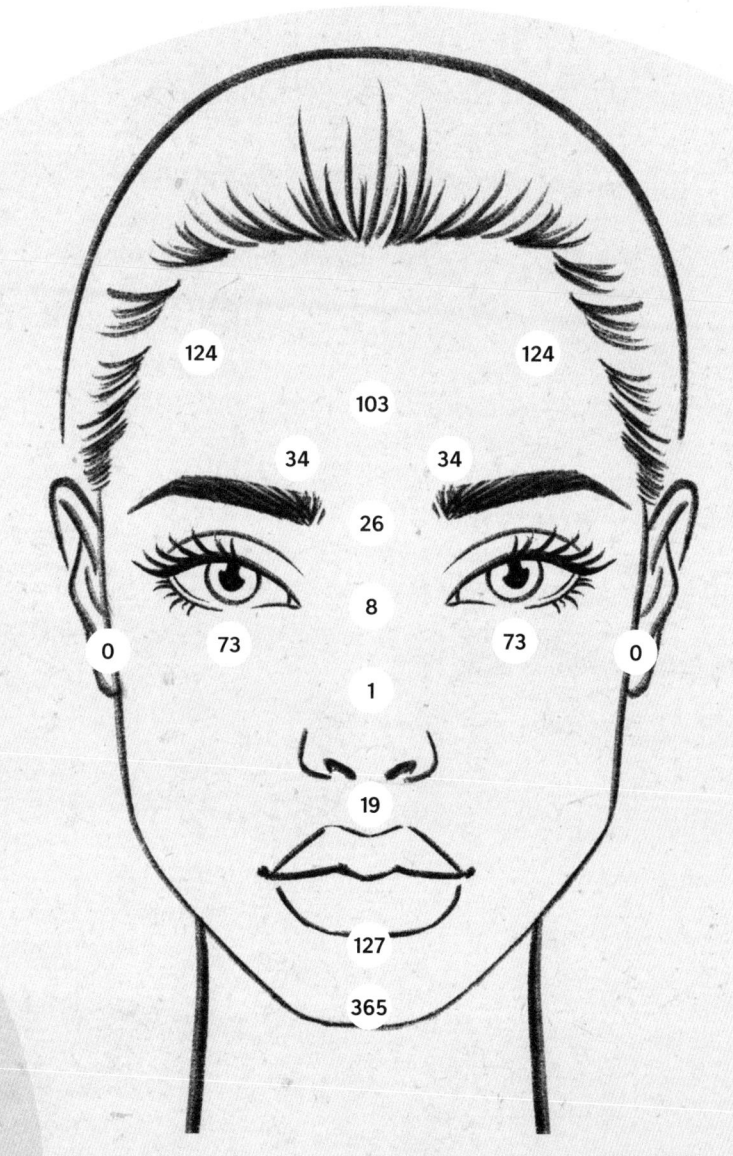

0: Reset and relax (see also page 48)
124: Brain, acne, depression, fatigue
103: Crown chakra, memory, fatigue
26: Third Eye chakra, eyes, neck
34: Shoulders, lungs, upper back
73: Lungs, kidneys, circulation

8: Throat chakra, coughs, temperature fluctuations and fever
1: Heart chakra, feeling cold, middle back
19: Solar Plexus chakra, colds, allergies
127: Sacral chakra, anxiety, exhaustion
365: Root chakra, lower back

eleven facial reflex zones 41

facial reflexology techniques

Reflexology movements are performed by simply putting varying degrees of pressure on the zones you wish to work on. You can apply this pressure with your fingers, a closed ballpoint pen, a reflexology wand, or any smooth, round-ended stick.

When working on reflex points or zones, the degree of pressure will vary according to the area you are working on and your general health. People with underlying health conditions often have very sensitive areas on their faces. You shouldn't try to hurt yourself in any way. If you find an area is particularly sensitive, ease the pressure and then increase it again as the pain subsides. If it doesn't get easier, move to an area close to the painful area and try pressing there instead.

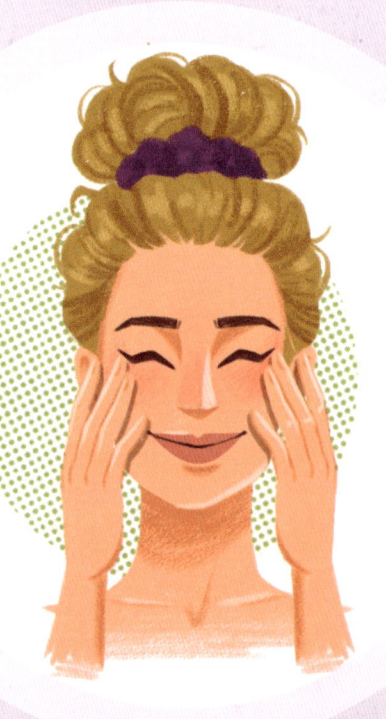

effleurage

Effleurage means "to skim" in French. When you train as a massage therapist, it is one of the first moves you learn, and in massage terms it means to stroke the skin. It is a slow, rhythmic, light movement to warm up the area you are working on.

tapping

I call this wonderfully relaxing and gently stimulating technique "raindrop fingers." It is done by gently tapping the index, middle, and ring fingers of both hands in a fluttering motion all over your face to create a rain-like effect. It can also be used as a warm-up for facial yoga (see page 17).

circles

Circles are made either with your index or middle fingers—you choose. First, press the reflex zone you are working on with one finger. Now make small, circular movements, but without moving from the spot, so you are moving your skin over the bone or cartilage, but not moving your finger over the skin.

pinching

I have included this movement because it is very relaxing and effective when used on the eyebrows. Simply make very light pinches with your thumbs and forefingers.

pressing

This is a classic facial reflexology technique, and it simply means pressing a reflex zone with a finger or reflexology tool. Pressure is usually held for a few seconds, released, and then repeated with varying degrees of pressure. Sometimes you might find that holding the pressure for longer will work better than taking the pressure on and off.

You can also move your fingers a little either up and down, diagonally, or side to side—use whichever feels best. As with the circles technique, you are moving your skin over the bone or cartilage and not moving your finger over the skin.

pressing and moving

If you are working on areas that reflect the spine, shoulders, or legs, you can do the pressing technique described above, but move along the zone—for example, up and down the nose or eyebrows.

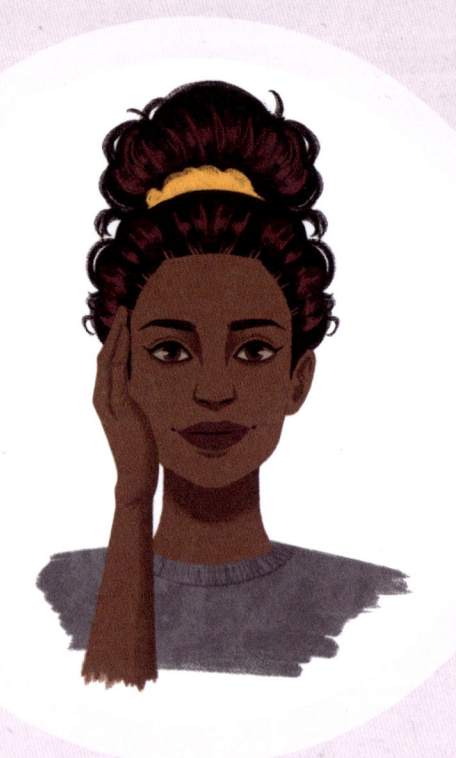

ear covering

When just one hand is being used to stimulate a reflex point, I like to cover the ear closest to my free hand in a shell-like fashion—cupped slightly and just lightly covering the ear. Each time only one hand is needed for a movement, I change the hand used for the movement and ear covering for the next zone, alternating the hands. This ear covering is wonderfully comforting, creating warmth and a slight whooshing noise.

The alternating of hands is great for left–right brain functioning, too. There are two hemispheres of the brain and a theory that people who are predominantly logical and analytical thinkers are left-brained, whereas right-brained people are said to be more artistic and free-thinking. By engaging both sides of the brain, we encourage a balanced attitude to life.

walking movement

A walking movement of the fingers and thumbs is used in foot reflexology, but it is not really suitable for the face. It is mentioned here as it is synonymous with reflexology in general.

TOOLS FOR FACIAL REFLEXOLOGY

One of the lovely things about facial reflexology is that you can do it with no tools other than your hands. However, it is fun to embellish your treatment with little luxuries such as:

•

A warm towel to place over your face at the beginning and/or end of your treatment.

•

Hydrosol (see page 92) to spritz over your face at the end of a treatment.

•

Facial oil (see page 96).

You may also wish to start using a reflexology wand that allows you to go deeper and be more precise once you feel confident in what you are doing.

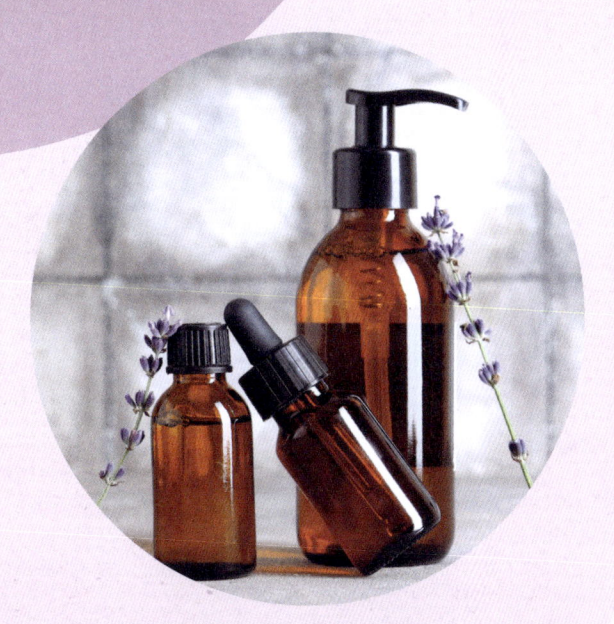

facial reflexology techniques   45

warm-up massage

I like to combine facial reflexology with a relaxing facial massage beforehand, which not only prepares the skin, but also creates a calm atmosphere.

For this warm-up massage, work from your forehead downward toward your chin for a relaxing effect. Downward massage of the face feels grounding and keeps you calm. The movements should be slow and rhythmical. (If you want to use this massage in the morning, work from the neck upward for a more invigorating effect, making the movements a little faster.)

1 Take a few lovely long, deep breaths before you begin this routine. Continue to keep your breathing slow and rhythmic throughout the routine. You may like to listen to music while performing the movements.

2 If you wish, apply a little facial oil (see page 96). This is not essential, but it works really well.

3 Use the tapping or "raindrop fingers" technique (see page 17), covering every part of your face in a symmetrical fashion. This also helps the oil sink in if you are using it.

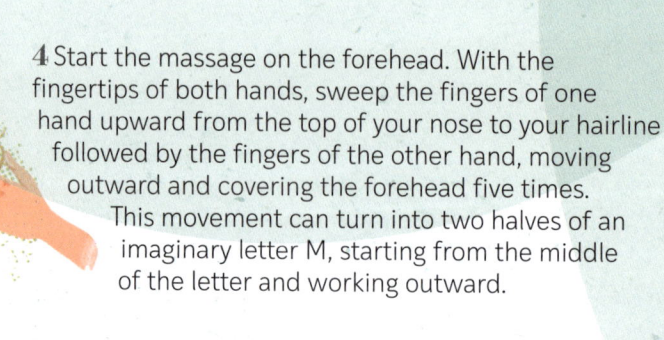

4 Start the massage on the forehead. With the fingertips of both hands, sweep the fingers of one hand upward from the top of your nose to your hairline followed by the fingers of the other hand, moving outward and covering the forehead five times. This movement can turn into two halves of an imaginary letter M, starting from the middle of the letter and working outward.

46 facial reflexology

5 Using your index and middle fingers, make circular movements on both of your temples at the same time, moving five times in one direction, then five times in the other direction, and taking care to move the skin and not move over the skin.

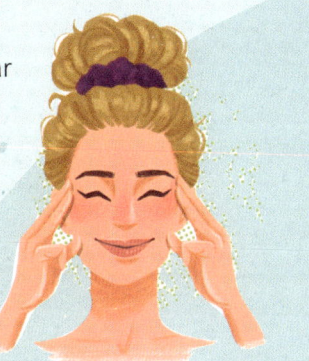

6 Using the thumb and index finger of both hands, lightly pinch the innermost part of both eyebrows for 5 seconds. Take off the pressure and move both hands out by about ½ inch (1 cm). Repeat until you reach the edges of your eyebrows. It should take about four pinches to cover your eyebrows. Repeat this process twice more.

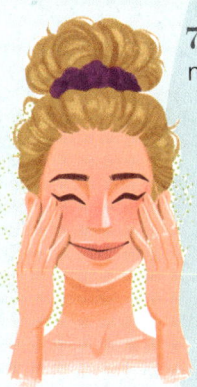

7 Place the index and middle fingers of both hands together at the bridge of your nose and slide them down and out, tracing the tops of your cheekbones five times.

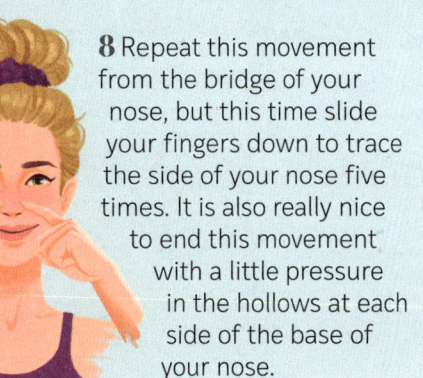

8 Repeat this movement from the bridge of your nose, but this time slide your fingers down to trace the side of your nose five times. It is also really nice to end this movement with a little pressure in the hollows at each side of the base of your nose.

9 Place your index and middle fingers on your fulcrum (the indentation below your nose and above your upper lip), then slide them out to the corner of your mouth as if you are drawing a moustache. Repeat five times.

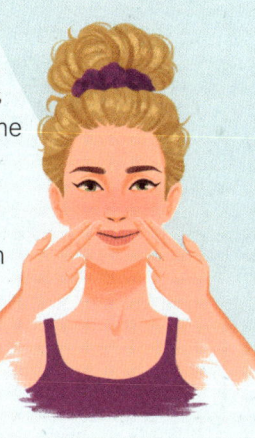

10 Place your middle fingers under your bottom lip, in the center, and then sweep them out to the corners of your lips five times, ending each movement with a little press at the corners of your mouth.

11 Place the backs of your fingers at the base of your neck and sweep them up to your chin. Repeat, working outward each time—five repetitions should cover your neck. Repeat the whole step four more times.

warm-up massage 47

five-minute evening routine

After doing the warm-up massage, this short facial reflexology routine will help you to relax physically and mentally, and also works on some of the chakras (see page 106). The routine might seem a little complicated on first reading, but it is incredibly simple once you have done it once or twice, so persevere!

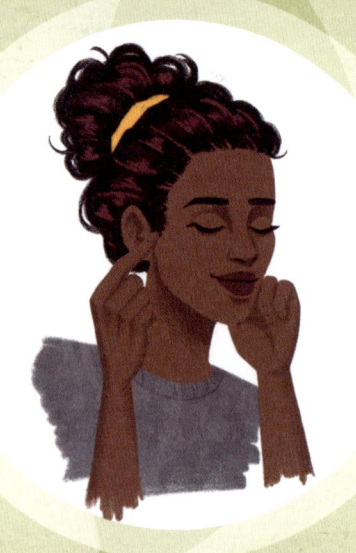

1 In facial reflexology, we always start and end a treatment at Zone 0, which is the Reset and Relax zone found close to your ears. Work on both sides at the same time by using your index fingers and pressing ten times.

2 Next, move to Zone 124, which is the Brain and Fatigue zone found on both sides of the top of your forehead. Use the pressing technique, moving back and forth diagonally about ½ inch (1 cm), to work on both sides at the same time, using your index fingers and pressing ten times.

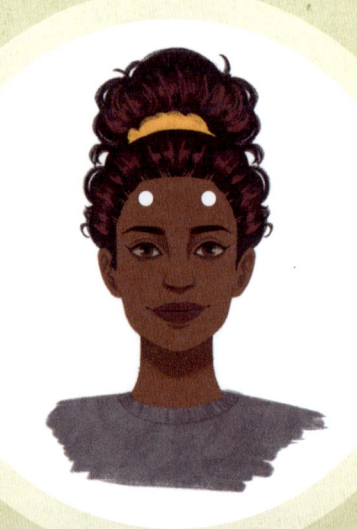

48 facial reflexology

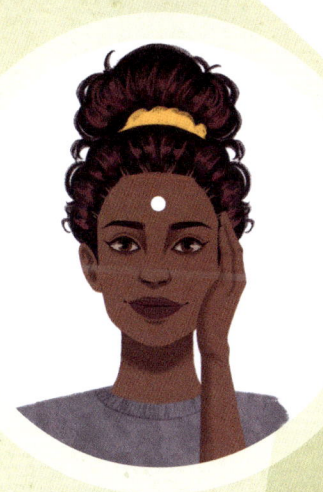

3 Put your left hand over your left ear and place the middle finger of your right hand on Zone 103, which is the Crown chakra, Memory, and Fatigue zone located right in the middle of your forehead. Make 10 circles counterclockwise.

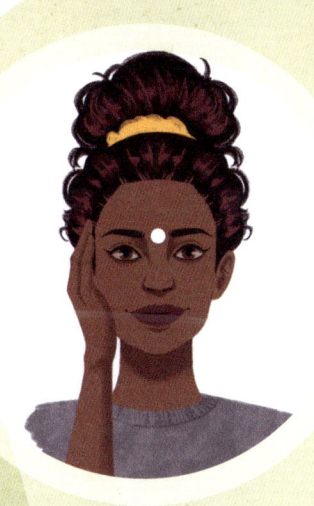

4 Now put your right hand over your right ear and place the middle finger of your left hand on Zone 26, which is the Third Eye, Eyes, and Neck zone located in between your eyebrows. Make 10 circles counterclockwise.

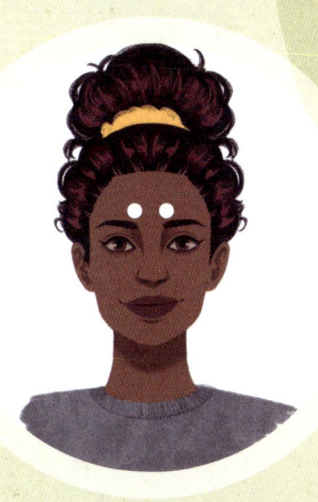

5 Working on both sides at the same time, using your index fingers, go to Zone 34, which is the Shoulders, Lungs, and Upper Back zone located just above your eyebrows, and press ten times.

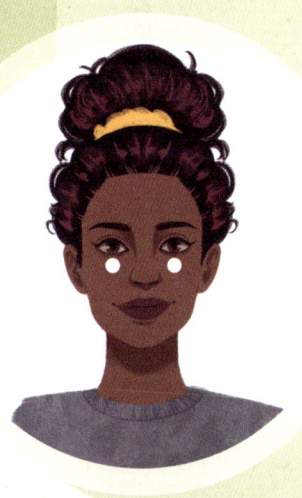

6 Working on both sides at the same time, using your index or middle fingers, whichever you prefer, move to Zone 73, which is the Lungs, Kidneys, and Circulation zone, located just under where your eye bags would be if you had them! Press ten times.

five-minute evening routine 49

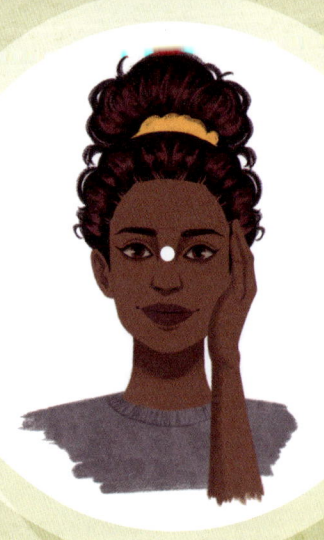

7 Place your left hand over your left ear and place the middle finger of your right hand on Zone 8, which is the Throat chakra, Coughs, and Temperature zone located right on the bridge of your nose. Make 10 circles counterclockwise.

8 While keeping your left hand over your left ear, move the middle finger of your right hand about ½ inch (1 cm) down your nose to Zone 1, which is the Heart, Feeling Cold, and Middle Back zone. Press ten times.

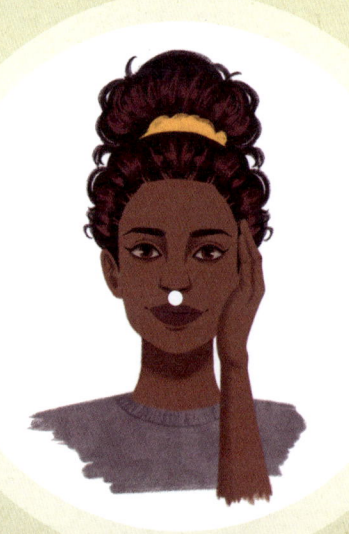

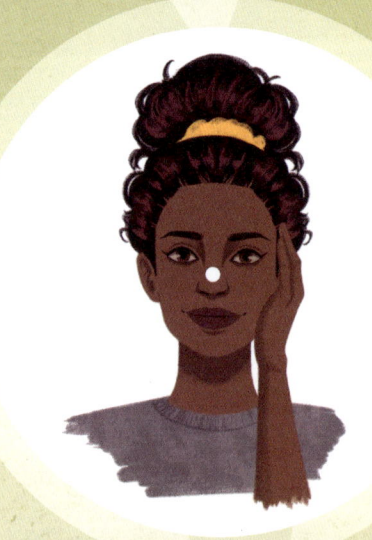

9 Still keeping your left hand over your left ear, move the middle finger of your right hand just below your nose to Zone 19, which is the Solar Plexus, Colds, and Allergies zone. Press ten times.

facial reflexology

10 Swap hands to place your right hand over your right ear and place the middle finger of your left hand just under your bottom lip on Zone 127, which is the Sacral chakra, Anxiety, and Exhaustion zone. Make 10 circles counterclockwise.

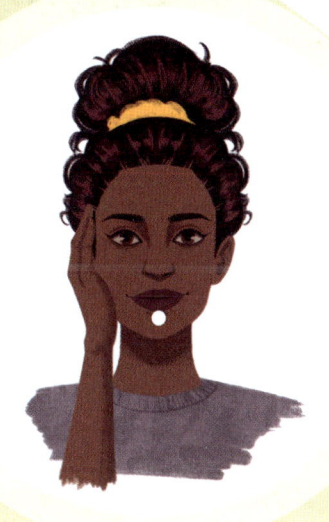

11 Still keeping your right hand over your right ear, move the middle finger of your left hand to Zone 365, which is the Root Chakra and Lower Back zone and is located on the dimple at the bottom of your chin. Make 10 circles counterclockwise.

12 Repeat Step 1 by pressing ten times on Zone 0, the Reset and Relax zone, to complete the sequence.

13 If desired, spritz a little hydrosol (see page 92) over your face, then cover your face with a warm towel, gently pressing it to your skin. Remove the towel and finish by taking a few deep breaths.

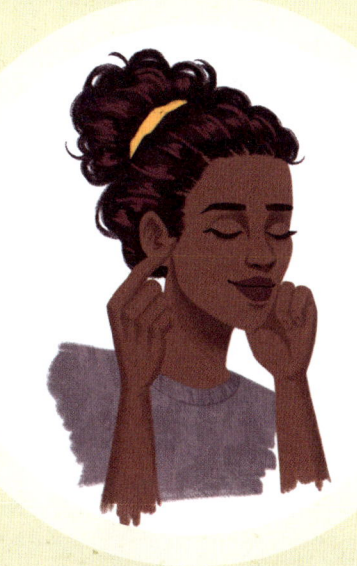

five-minute evening routine

facial mapping

Facial mapping, also known as mien shiang, is a 3,000-year-old system of diagnosing conditions of the body reflected in the face. It stems from Traditional Chinese Medicine and Ayurvedic medicine.

Facial mapping works on the same principles as facial reflexology in that energy or qi can become blocked, causing imbalances in the body. These imbalances can show up on the face in many ways—breakouts, redness, dryness, oiliness, lines, puffiness, wrinkles, deep lines, and other anomalies that might appear. It utilizes broader, larger areas than the reflex zones or points used in facial reflexology.

Even though facial mapping is a largely unproven method of diagnosis, its findings over thousands of years have withstood time and are based on often obvious but not necessarily recognized signs. A spotty or pimply chin, for instance, indicates hormonal fluctuations and an imbalance in the reproductive system. These kinds of pimples and spots nearly always appear in teenagers and menopausal women—the time when hormones are on the rampage.

In more modern versions of facial mapping, such as acne face mapping which has become very popular, signals on the face can be attributed to things like pillows, cell phones, makeup brushes, or flannels needing to be sanitized or replaced, or products not agreeing with your skin, which makes perfect sense. Even though this sounds obvious and hardly an ancient diagnostic technique, it stays with the principle of noticing and reading what you see in someone's face.

Whichever way you look at it, facial mapping can be a great tool to direct you toward small changes that might make the world of difference to how fresh and healthy you look and feel. Practitioners of facial mapping usually use it in addition to other practices like facial yoga and facial reflexology as a way to monitor imbalances in the body and a quick method to see progress. It is helpful to understand facial mapping for yourself, too, in order to know exactly when you might need to make some minor changes to your habits before they turn into something more troublesome.

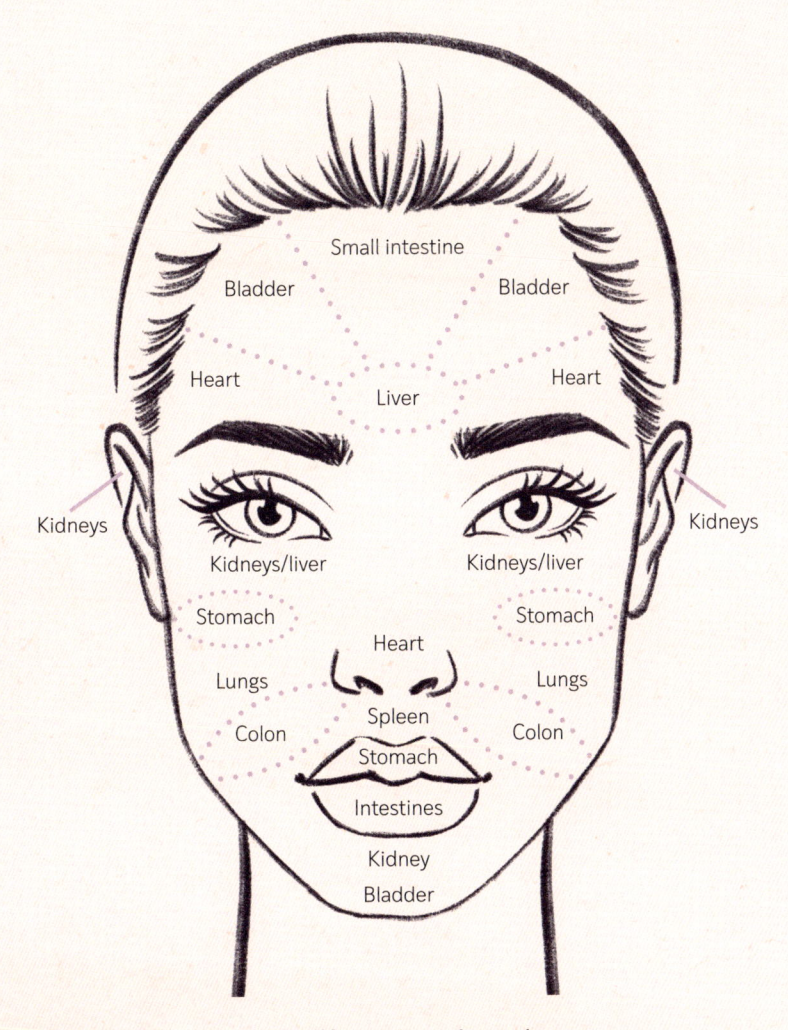

mind–body integration

The image above shows a Traditional Chinese Medicine version of facial mapping. Unlike the facial reflexology chart on page 39, it only shows the organs.

facial mapping 53

organs and emotions

Taking this concept a little deeper, in Traditional Chinese Medicine, our organs and our emotions are intertwined, so our emotions can affect our organs, and vice versa. So, if you find that a certain area of your face is displaying some of the symptoms mentioned on page 52 or doesn't look quite right, you could consult the circles below to find out which emotions are connected with the organ that area represents to see if that helps.

heart
When in balance reflects
joy

When unbalanced reflects
deep sadness

lungs
When in balance reflects
happiness

When unbalanced reflects
sorrow/grief

stomach
When in balance reflects
courage

When unbalanced reflects
fear

spleen
When in balance reflects
thought

When unbalanced reflects
negativity

liver
When in balance reflects
love

When unbalanced reflects
anger

gallbladder
When in balance reflects
decisiveness

When unbalanced reflects
indecisiveness/ bitterness

large intestine

When in balance reflects **security**

When unbalanced reflects **fear/anxiety**

kidneys

When in balance reflects **trust**

When unbalanced reflects **fear/worry**

bladder

When in balance reflects **peace/calm**

When unbalanced reflects **stress/resentment**

pancreas

When in balance reflects **security**

When unbalanced reflects **shock**

small intestine

When in balance reflects **clarity**

When unbalanced reflects **confusion**

thyroid

When in balance reflects **sociability/gregariousness**

When unbalanced reflects **solitude/reclusiveness**

contact dermatitis

Many people develop various levels of contact dermatitis (also known as touch dermatitis) on their face, which is a form of eczema caused by contact with something that aggravates your skin, such as chemicals in products or even just dust. Often it gets worse as your fingers subconsciously return to an area time and time again, causing redness, soreness, and sometimes itchiness.

If this is happening to you, in addition to consulting a health professional, you could see which organ and emotion that the area you are returning to represents and adjust your thoughts and habits accordingly.

A quick fix to stop yourself continually touching the troublesome area is to keep some natural balm or oil which contains either tea tree or lavender essential oil close by. Apply it to your fingertips regularly, so it creates a reminder and therapeutic barrier.

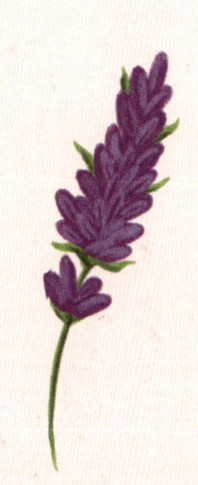

facial mapping

CHAPTER 3

gua sha and cryotherapy

Facial massage is not only supremely relaxing, but it also brings blood to the area being worked on by stimulating circulation—which, in turn, gives the skin a brighter complexion. By using gua sha or cryotherapy, you can increase the effectiveness of your massage.

what is gua sha?

Gua sha is the practice of using tools to massage your face, rather than just your fingers, which can improve circulation and therefore your complexion.

Gua sha is an ancient technique that began in Asia thousands of years ago. As with reflexology, it was an alternative treatment to acupuncture and was used to treat pain, inflammation, and immunity deficiencies in the body by clearing channels and venting heat through the skin, similar to the way sweating can expel toxins. The use of gua sha causes heat and varying degrees of redness on the area being treated from repetitive rubbing. This heat can last for many days after a treatment, which can be a great pain reliever.

Gua sha is still used holistically for the treatment of conditions all over the body, usually as an extension of massage, but nowadays it is also hailed as a beauty treatment, and all sorts of tools are available for use in beauty spas and at home (see page 60). Using gua sha on the face is very different to when it is being used on the body for injuries and strains where it is a deep and sometimes painful experience. When performed on the face either at home or in a beauty spa or clinic, it is very gentle, but it still produces great results.

how does gua sha work?

This treatment is not like facial yoga, which builds and tones the muscles of your face, or facial reflexology, which affects your whole body, sometimes quite profoundly. Gua sha can have an instant effect, which is very satisfying.

Let's look at what gua sha means:
- *Gua* means to "rub" or "scrape."
- *Sha* means "red" or "skin rash."

It may not sound like a very attractive activity, but the principle is that by rubbing the skin red, it can purge the skin and body of impurities and problems large or small.

In practice, this means gua sha can offer a natural instant face lift. This is because it can improve the flow and drainage of lymph (the fluid that flows through the body), which removes stagnant toxins and reduces puffiness, and can make you look brighter, fresher, and more awake.

Other benefits include:
- Stimulating the production of collagen, which can make your skin look firmer.
- Helping to smooth fascia, a layer of connective tissue found below the skin. When fascia is gently stressed by gua sha, it can tighten up, giving your face a firmer look.
- Lessening scars by disrupting and smoothing out scar tissue.
- Reducing muscular knots, especially those around the jawline caused by clenching your teeth, by encouraging them to relax.

what is cryotherapy?

While gua sha produces heat and redness, cryotherapy means cold therapy. Coldness can decrease inflammation by constricting blood vessels, which slows circulation to the area being cooled. It works in much the same way as icing an injury. Cryotherapy is great for a quick fix to lessen puffiness and to give you an instant pick-me-up.

choosing your tools

Originally, gua sha would have been performed with a Chinese soup spoon, a piece of sacred animal bone, or even buffalo horns. Nowadays, there are myriad beautiful tools to use for your gua sha.

Scrapers and rollers are the most common gua sha tools:

- Rollers (below left) are intended to cover larger areas such as your cheeks, forehead, and neck. Rollers work best for drainage and detox, because you can make light, repetitive strokes. Lymphatic drainage and any kind of detox requires patience as you need to work on these areas regularly and results will only show after a few days or even weeks of practicing gua sha daily. Don't be in a rush and keep it gentle for the best results.
- Scrapers (below right) are used for contouring the jaw and cheekbones. They are usually smooth, flat, and heart-shaped, but they may also be ridged and comb-like. They work best for a cosmetic lift, because you can apply more pressure with them.

There are many other types of gua sha tools. It is good to be at one with your gua sha tool, so you might find you collect a few different types, but instinctively return to one more than the others. Your tool needs to nestle comfortably in your hand and glide easily over the contours of your face and neck.

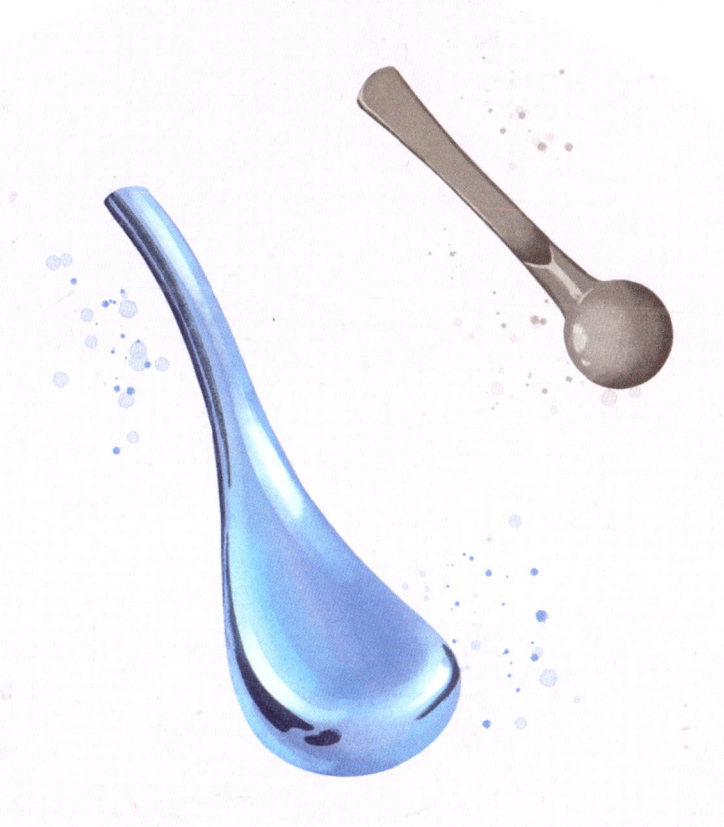

cryotherapy tools

Cryotherapy balls or globes (above left) are usually used as a pair, so you work all over your face with a tool in each hand. They are usually metal, so they stay cold by themselves, but they can be placed in the fridge for a real cryo experience. When working with cool or cold tools, you should keep the treatment very light and gentle, especially as these tools are often used for puffiness under the eyes. Small metal roller balls (above right) are super soothers for tired eyes. Cryo tools are also good to have on hand during the day, as their coolness can give you a nice wakeup boost.

choosing your tools

types of natural stones used for gua sha tools

Natural stone or crystal gua sha tools are most often made from rose quartz or jade. If you search a little harder, you will find gua sha tools made from other natural stones too. You might find that you are drawn to a specific color or look. Each type of stone has its own significance, properties, and energy, which adds another lovely layer of consciousness and intention to your gua sha self-treatment.

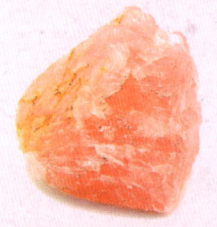

Rose quartz is associated with the Heart chakra (see page 106) and gives a feeling of love, healing, peace, and calm.

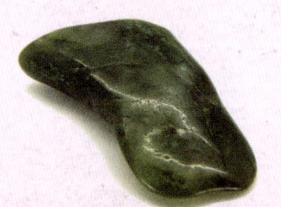

Green jade gives a sense of security, resilience, and prosperity. It is balancing and strengthening. It is also associated with positivity.

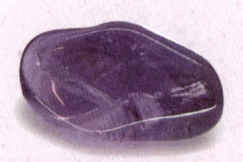

Amethyst is soothing and calming. It can also help with inflammation.

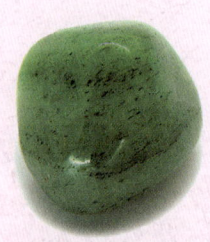

Aventurine is lucky and calming.

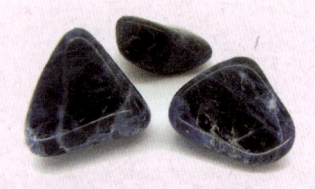

Sodalite helps relieve tension and imparts focus.

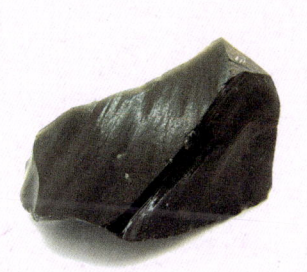

Obsidian helps detox and strengthen skin that is undernourished.

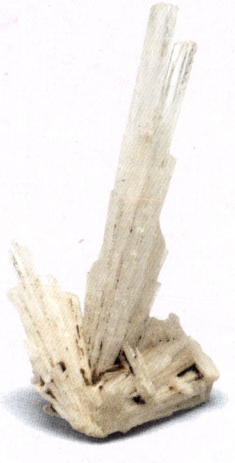

Scolecite creates a peaceful atmosphere.

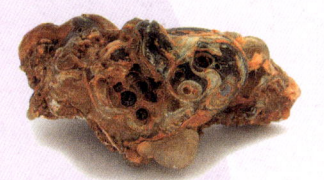

Fire agate makes you feel courageous and passionate. (It is not very easy to find gua sha tools made of fire agate, but they do exist if you search!)

TAKING CARE OF YOUR TOOLS

Don't keep your gua sha tools in the bottom of a drawer! You need to have them on hand, so that you use them often.

•

Keep your tools in a bag when not in use.

•

Always make sure your gua sha tools are clean and crack- and chip-free. The tools are robust, so should remain intact if dropped, but check them before using and wash them if they have been on the floor.

•

Wash your tools with warm, soapy water after each use, and dry them carefully.

how to gua sha

On pages 68–69 there is a full gua sha routine you can try, but it is helpful to keep the following points in mind as a general guide.

Using a gua sha tool couldn't really be any easier. Simply sweep the gua sha tool across the area you are working on, and repeatedly massage until the skin becomes a little pink.

Use whichever part of the tool fits the contours of your face best:

- A long, smooth edge of a scraper tool works well on larger areas like the cheeks and neck.
- Bends or crook shapes in heart-shaped scrapers work well along the jawline, with one side above and one below the jaw.
- Shorter edges or small rollers work well on smaller areas such as the forehead and mouth.

Make your movements firm, but not hard. Light repetition is best to achieve a pink glow. Always err on the side of caution—less can be more. A gentle massage with a gua sha tool will still give great results. Never push the tool into your face.

Speed doesn't really matter either. Slow is more relaxing, but sometimes you might want to speed up the movements to complete the massage more quickly or perhaps to make it more invigorating.

Work in one direction, not back and forth. Make a sweep, lift the tool, and repeat. Try to get into a rhythm. This can be an opportunity for a meditative moment.

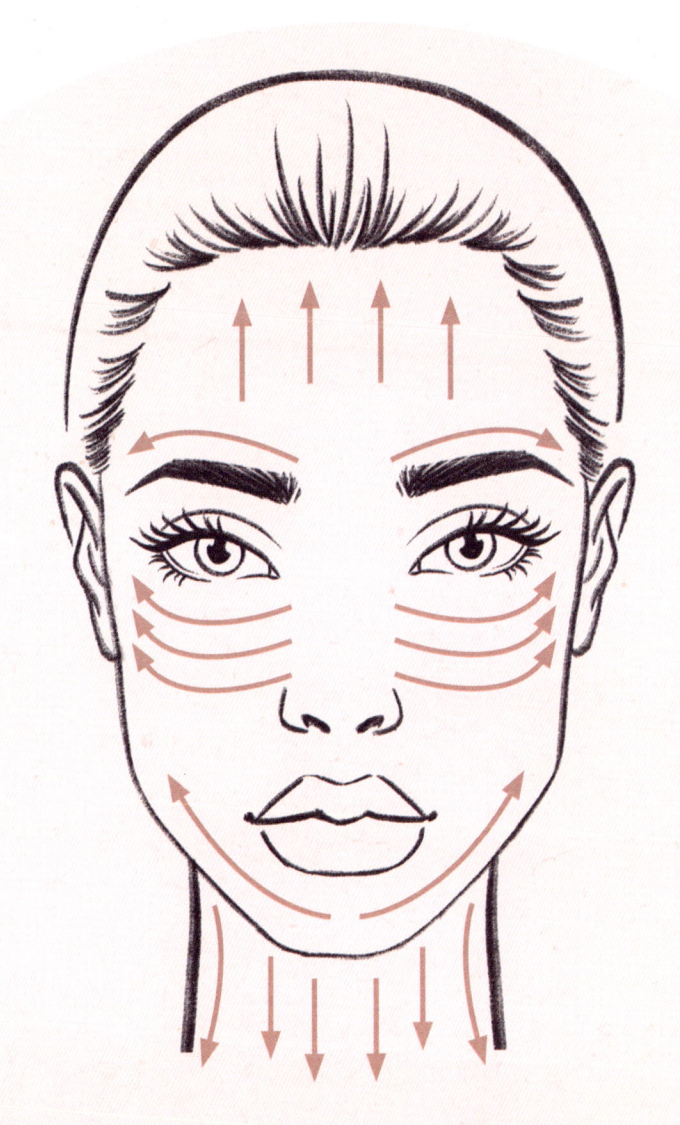

gua sha directions

This simple chart shows the areas and directions for a gua sha massage, which can be done with a roller or scraper. This is just a starting point: you will develop your own contours to work along as you use your tool more, and the chart could show many more arrows to reflect this, but it would become unclear. Unlike acupuncture and reflexology, you don't need to work to specific points or zones. The only real rule is to work outward from the nose, not inward. If you were to try an inward movement, you would know why you shouldn't do it—it will crinkle up the skin and feel very uncomfortable. A gua sha massage should be a relaxing, meditative, and rejuvenating experience.

You will notice that the arrows on the neck go down, rather than up. Most beauty massages work upward and outward, which is the natural way, as, after all, we want our faces and neck to look fresh, not saggy. However, as previously explained, gua sha is brilliant for lymphatic drainage, which helps reduce swelling, and so we work downward toward the lymph nodes. The movement from just behind the ears to your collarbone feels particularly lovely as this activates the vagus nerve (see page 102).

CAUTIONS FOR FACIAL GUA SHA

Only use your tools on clean, unbroken skin. Do not gua sha on broken or recently injured skin.

•

Even though gua sha is sometimes called "scraping," do not scrape the skin. Your tool should glide effortlessly over your skin.

•

Do not gua sha if you have type 1 diabetes or circulatory problems, or if you take blood thinning medication.

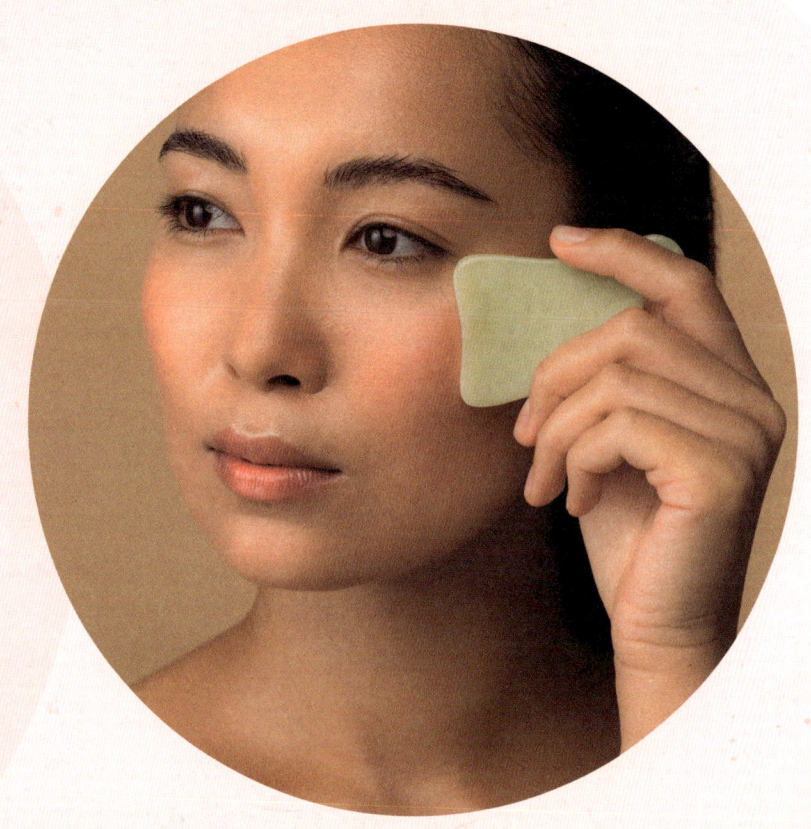

when to use gua sha

Timewise, there is no specific time to gua sha, but personally I find it best in the morning. Two or three times per week is sufficient to make a difference, but if you build it into your routine with just a few moves each day, you will see the change in the tone and definition of your face more quickly.

If you work at a desk, you can keep a gua sha tool nearby and use it to relieve tension in your shoulders or forearms from typing.

should I use gua sha or cryotherapy?

Gua sha works best if you are looking to improve the texture of your skin and iron out knots and scar tissue. Cryotherapy is best for soothing distressed skin and for reducing puffiness.

gua sha routine

For this routine, I suggest using a heart-shaped scraper as it allows you to cover all contours of the face.

1 Cleanse your face as you would normally.

2 If you wish, spritz your face with a hydrosol (see page 92).

3 Apply 5 drops of oil. This can be a favorite facial oil (see page 96) or a single plant oil (see pages 78–83). You only need enough oil to allow the gua sha tool to slide across the skin without dragging (you don't want an oil slick!), so add a little more if your skin absorbs it too quickly.

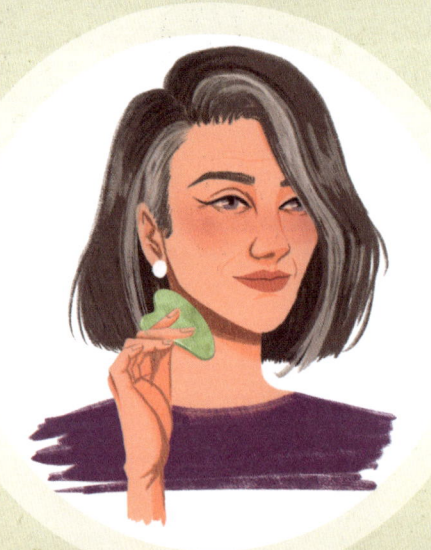

4 Start the gua sha routine by using the side of your tool to rub gently from behind your right ear down in a gentle diagonal toward your shoulder blade. Repeat this move eight times: eight usually fits in with music, if you are listening to it, so you can do this rhythmically. Repeat on the other side.

5 Using the side of the tool, rub gently from under your chin down toward your décolletage and work outward toward one ear, then repeat from the centerline to the other ear. Four downward strokes will cover each side, so you will make eight strokes in total to cover the whole neck. Repeat four times. This will help to drain away toxins by encouraging them toward lymph nodes.

6 Using the bend in the tool, start in the middle of your chin and trace your jawline out eight times to one side, then repeat on the other side.

68 gua sha and cryotherapy

7 Using the side of the tool, rub along one of your cheeks below the cheekbone eight times, then repeat on the other side.

8 Using one of the shorter edges of the tool, repeat step 7 much more gently above your cheekbones.

9 Using the shortest edge of the tool, rub from just above the tip of your nose out to one side of your nose eight times, then repeat on the other side.

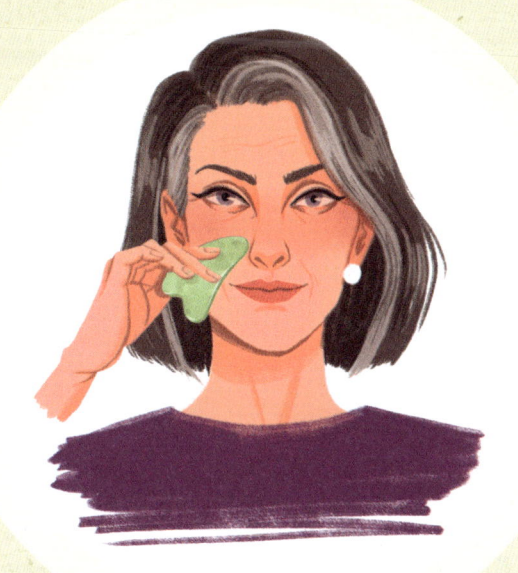

10 Continuing with a short edge, rub from the center of your eyebrows outward to one side over your forehead, just above the eyebrows, eight times. Repeat on the other side.

11 Now rub upward from the eyebrows over the rest of your forehead eight times with whichever of the shorter edges of the tool feels most comfortable.

12 Rub any area that feels as if it needs a little more work or that you may have missed out.

13 If you wish, end with another spritz of hydrosol.

TOP TIP

When switching sides, you can also switch the hand you are using to hold your gua sha tool if this is easy for you or if it feels right. Switching hands is good for your left–right brain activity, but for actual gua sha benefits it is not necessary. If you find it easier, use just one hand for all steps.

cryotherapy routine

For this sequence you will need a pair of cryo balls, so you can hold one in each hand and work on both sides of your face at the same time.

1 Cleanse your face as you would normally.

2 If you wish, spritz your face with a hydrosol (see page 92).

3 Apply 5 drops of oil. This can be a favorite facial oil (see page 96) or a single plant oil (see pages 78–83). You only need enough oil to allow the cryo tool to slide across the skin without dragging (you don't want an oil slick!), so add a little more if your skin absorbs it too quickly.

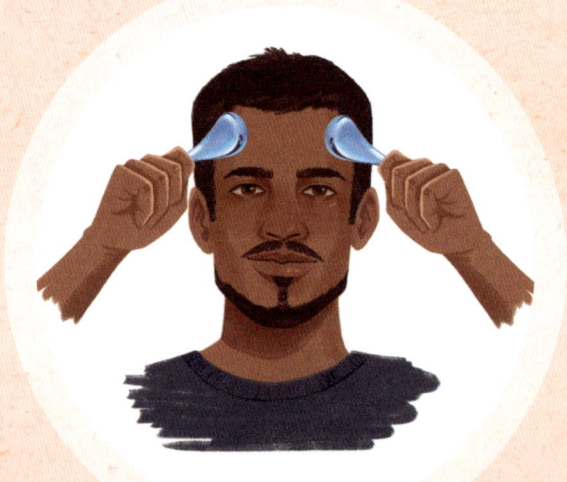

4 Start by gliding the tools eight times from the center of your forehead out toward your temples.

5 Glide the tools eight times from the center of your eyebrows outward across your eyebrows.

6 Sweep the tools eight times very gently under your eyes, from the center of your face outward, to reduce any puffiness.

7 Sweep the tools eight times under your cheekbones, from the center of your face outward.

gua sha and cryotherapy

8 Sweep the tools eight times above your lip from the center to the corners of your mouth.

9 Sweep the tools eight times from under your bottom lip right up to your ears.

10 Sweep the tools eight times along your jawline, working from the center out, starting gently on the bone and slipping off it toward the neck as if you are sculpting your jawline. You may want to use the tools to massage the back of your jaw near your ear where you might grind your teeth a little. This can be especially satisfying.

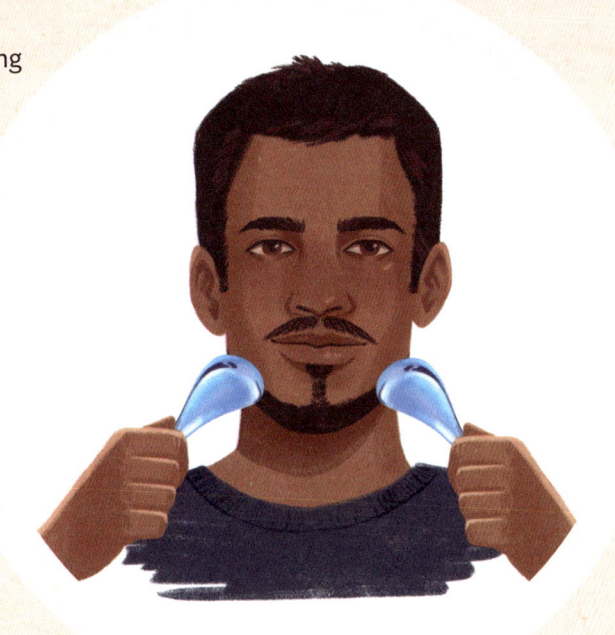

11 Sweep the tools from under your chin down toward your décolletage and work out toward one ear, then repeat from the centerline to the other ear. Four downward strokes will cover each side, so you will make eight strokes in total to cover the whole neck.

12 If you wish, end with a little spritz of hydrosol.

cryotherapy routine 71

CHAPTER 4

recipes for super skin

Facial reflexology and gua sha are much more effective when performed with plant oils, which are natural and readily available, and which can also form part of your general skincare routine. When you add carefully selected essential oils to plant oils, you can create a spa experience at home with all the therapeutic benefits that these have to offer.

why ditch the chemicals?

An average of 64 percent of what you put on your skin is absorbed into your body. With that in mind, it's vital to consider what is really in products that seem so appealing.

All creams and lotions contain synthetic preservatives, emulsifiers, or bulking agents. Preservatives are designed to kill all bacteria—but this includes the vital bacteria that form the protective microbial outer layer of our skin. Emulsifiers, the detergents of skincare ingredients, bind oil and water together and strip your skin of natural oil, leaving it gasping for elasticity and producing yet more oil, which is often the reason for oily outbreaks. Bulking agents such as cornstarch, lactose, sucrose, and glycine, used to affect the texture and increase the volume of some products, can clog the skin, stopping it from breathing while causing blackheads and spots. There is always a product to correct the one that is doing the harm, and another to correct that one, and voilà: a multimillion-dollar industry is in motion.

waterless skincare

Waterless skincare, as the name suggests, refers to products formulated without water and containing only plant oils and waxes. The absence of water means that bacteria cannot grow in these products, so harsh preservatives are not required. It is sometimes called conscious, ethical, or, of course, natural skincare.

Water is vital for life and it is important to conserve it. Billions of gallons of water are used unnecessarily in the manufacturing of most skincare products. A cream typically contains around 65 percent water and a lotion contains 80 percent. Waterless skincare is more concentrated and therefore more effective. Plus, shipping large amounts of water around the world also wastes a huge amount of energy. Imagine how much smaller waterless shipments of skincare are, and how much water is therefore being saved.

Water in skincare is completely unnecessary. Don't let people tell you that your skin needs "hydration"—our skin is designed to keep the inside of our bodies dry! Yes, it draws water from the lower dermis and from humectants (ingredients that attract water to the skin) in skincare products, but natural humectants, such as jojoba and sunflower oils, work brilliantly because they do not evaporate quickly on the skin as many creams and lotions do.

There are some exceptions, though. Hydrolats, more commonly known as hydrosols, are a by-product of the extraction process of essential oils and some other ingredients, and they retain many of the properties of the plants they came from. These waters are often used alone for their therapeutic properties and are ethical in that they would otherwise be thrown away. Hydrosols do not contain preservatives because they are packed with natural antibacterial properties, meaning that they do not strip our skin of its natural goodness. We will find out more about hydrosols on page 92.

The great news is that large skincare corporations are investing heavily in developing more natural and waterless ranges, which include balms, oils, solid shampoos, and cleansers, to name just a few. Meanwhile, there are thousands of small independent beauty companies waving the banner of healthy, conscious, and ethical skincare. (See Resources, page 125.)

You can start your natural skincare journey by using simple plant oils individually or by mixing them together yourself following my guidelines on the following pages.

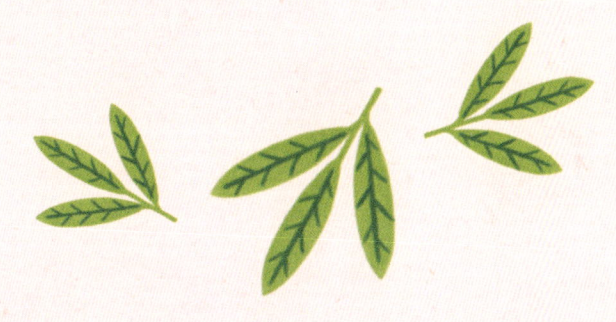

why ditch the chemicals?

what are plant oils and essential oils?

If you want to make the shift toward natural skincare, it is important to learn about the different types of oils and how they can be used.

Plant oils are oils and waxes that are extracted from plants. Other names used for plant oils are base/carrier oils, fruit oils, vegetable oils, and macerated or infused oils. Plant oils are not only used in skincare. They are also used in cooking, cleaning, medicine, animal care, machinery, and cosmetics. You can find out more about the plant oils used in skincare on pages 78–83.

Essential oils are also derived from plants but are not actually oily. They are volatile extracts, which means they are extremely delicate and evaporate easily, so need to be extracted, stored, and handled with care.

There are many ways to extract oils from plants. These include cold pressing, steam distillation, enfleurage, expression, carbon dioxide extraction, and solvent extraction, among others.

MINERAL OILS

In many cosmetic and body-care products, mineral oils are also used, but these are not ideal for skincare. Mineral oils are extracted from the earth, so you could call them "natural," but they are not environmentally friendly because they are not renewable by the earth. They are also not absorbed easily by the skin. Rather than moisturizing the deeper layers of the epidermis (the surface layer of the skin, made up of five layers itself), they tend to create a barrier, locking in any germs that might be there and stopping the skin from breathing.

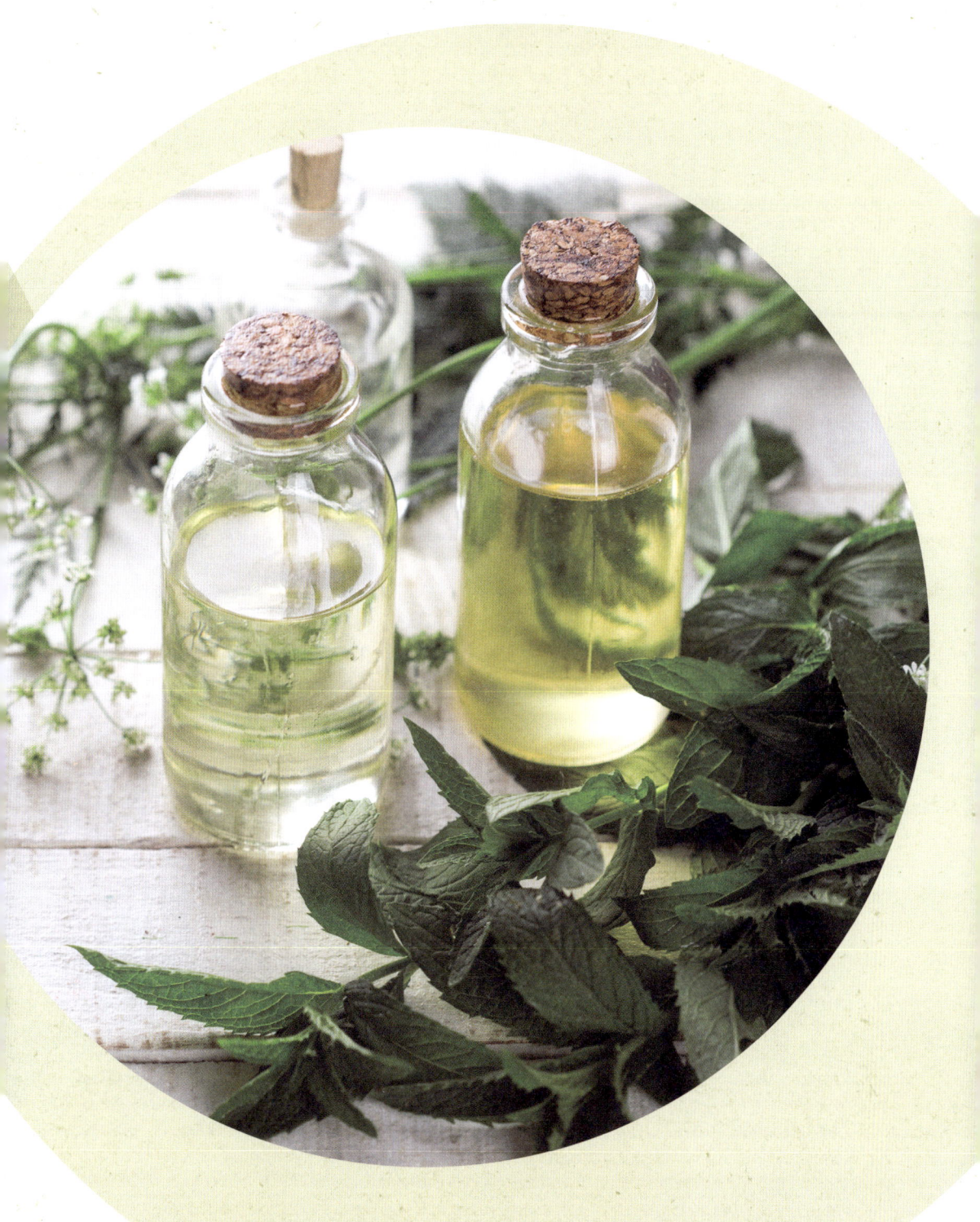

what are plant oils and essential oils?

base oils

Base oils, also known as carrier oils, used to be just that—used mostly as a base for more active and concentrated essential oils to in effect "dilute" them. Now, though, we are far more knowledgeable about what they are capable of.

Base oils come in many different weights: some are thick and viscous, described as heavyweight; some are lightweight; and some are mediumweight. Some are more easily absorbed by the skin than others. They can be antioxidant or antiviral, and they can help to smooth fine lines or even regulate oil secretion. Their possibilities are endless.

how to use base oils

Base oils can be used individually or combined with each other to achieve a rich, medium, or lightweight moisturizer which is mostly fragrance free. (Some base oils do have a slight natural fragrance.) For example, if you are using coconut oil, which is lightweight, you might want to add some jojoba oil, which is heavyweight, to thicken it up. Some oils also work well as cleansers.

For facial massage, lightweight base oils allow your fingers or gua sha/cryo tools to glide across your skin more easily. The addition of richer oils, such as jojoba or argan oil, will make your massage more nourishing.

There are very few precautions to adhere to with base oils. Base oils used on their own are super safe. However, if you have a nut allergy, you may want to steer clear of nut-based oils, such as sweet almond oil; they are rarely a problem, but consult a professional before using.

coconut oil *Caprylic/capric triglyceride*; **lightweight**

Virgin coconut oil is solid until it is warmed up to turn it to liquid, and returns to its solid state again once cooled. Therefore, to make a face oil, we use fractionated coconut oil, which means the fatty part of the oil has been removed, making the oil liquid at all temperatures. This process makes the oil odorless, but it also prolongs its shelf life.

I like to use fractionated coconut oil as a light cleanser. It easily dissolves makeup and can be wiped away with a damp cloth or flannel. It also has antibacterial properties, which makes it ideal for cleansing.

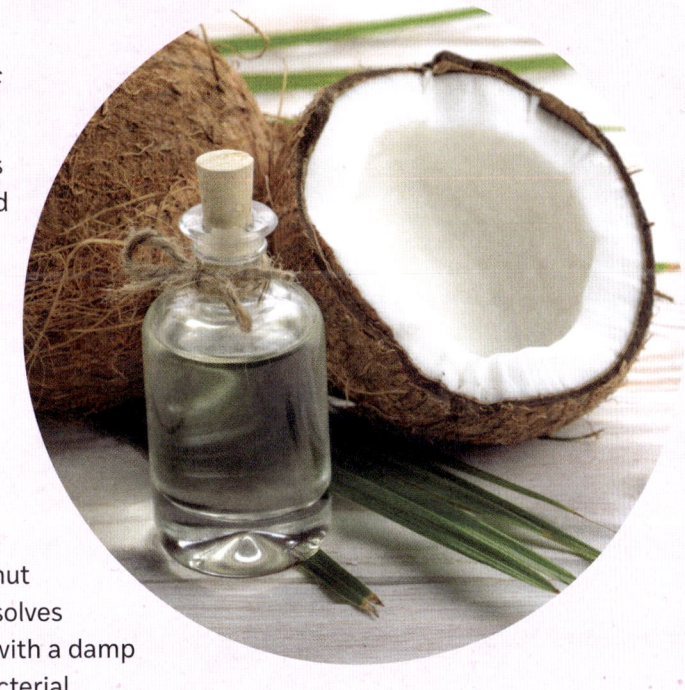

peach kernel oil *Prunus persica*; **lightweight**

As the name suggests, this oil derives from the kernel (pit or seed) of peaches.

Peach kernel oil is rich in beta-carotene, an antioxidant that converts to vitamin A in the body, and vitamin E. It is a light, non-greasy, and highly emollient oil that is very nourishing for dry skin.

Peach kernel oil is also hypoallergenic, so it is ideal for those with sensitive skin. It is easily absorbed, has good penetration, and leaves no oily residue or greasy feeling on the skin.

base oils

vitamin E oil *Tocopherol*; lightweight as an infusion

In this oil, a base oil—usually sunflower oil (*Helianthus annuus*)—is infused with vitamin E, which not only helps to prolong the life of the oil but is also wonderful for treating scars and blemishes.

Vitamin E protects the cells and cell membranes from free-radical and environmental oxidative stress. The vitamin is normally found in the skin, but exposure to sunlight has been shown to deplete this extremely important antioxidant, so applying it topically can boost its availability. Adequate levels of tocopherol become increasingly important in mature skin as it has been shown to decrease with age.

As well as its antioxidant properties, vitamin E is required for healthy collagen in the skin – which is the skin's support system and helps it remain firm and healthy. It also helps to moisturize the skin and even more importantly aids tissue repair, thereby keeping the skin in good condition. In tests, it was found that a solution containing 5 percent of vitamin E applied to wounds decreased the healing time required and helped stop the wound reopening.

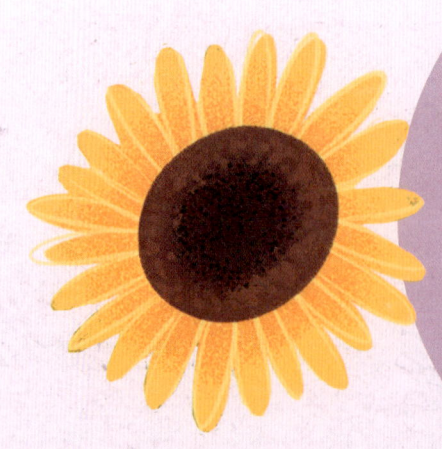

INFUSIONS AND MACERATIONS

When you see that an oil is infused or macerated, this is a base oil, such as sunflower oil, which has had herbs or flowers infused into it to harness their therapeutic properties in oil form. Herbs such as *Calendula* are often used for infusions, as is vitamin E. Most infusions are lightweight oils, because sunflower is a lightweight oil.

calendula oil *Calendula officinalis;* **lightweight**

Calendula oil is usually made with sunflower oil (*Helianthus annuus*) which has been infused with *Calendula officinalis*. Calendula has been used for centuries for ornamental purposes, as well as culinary, cosmetic, and medicinal reasons. *Calendula officinalis* is similar to other marigolds (*Tagetes*) and is often called by the alternative name pot marigold.

Calendula contains flavonoids, which give it strong anti-inflammatory properties, and a high concentration of linoleic acid. This acid gives calendula oil powerful antimicrobial and antiviral properties.

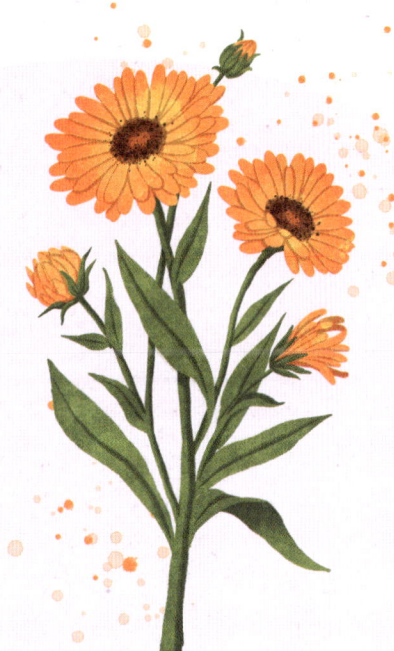

argan oil *Argania spinosa;* **mediumweight**

Inside the fruit of the argan tree is a little nut that gives us argan oil. For generations, natives of the Argan Forest in Morocco have pressed the nut to extract this precious oil to use to heal wounds, relieve rashes, and nourish skin and hair. These slow-growing trees are so revered that in 1998 the Argan Forest was declared a Biosphere Reserve by UNESCO.

Argan oil is now used all over the world as a natural moisturizer for skin and hair and to treat skin infections, bug bites, and skin rashes. It is absorbed quickly and does not leave an oily residue.

One of the main reasons that argan oil is so healing is that it is not only packed with antioxidants, omega-6 fatty acids, and linoleic acid, but is also rich in vitamins: vitamin A helps to reduce fine wrinkles while keeping delicate skin moisturized, and vitamin E helps to boost cell production while promoting healthy skin and hair. Research shows that when applied to skin, argan oil also eases inflammation.

rosehip oil *Rosa canina*; **mediumweight**

Rosehip oil is rich in vitamin A, which helps to prevent premature aging caused by sun exposure. When skin is exposed to the sun, it can increase levels of enzymes that lead to the breakdown of collagen and elastin. Rosehip oil can help combat this.

Antioxidants are micronutrients that protect tissues in the body and rosehip oil is rich in antioxidants, including beta-carotene and lycopene. These help to protect and repair skin from premature aging caused by modern living.

Aging causes skin collagen fibers to fragment or break down. Essential fatty acids play a key role in the maintenance and regeneration of the collagen and elastin fibers that keep skin firm and youthful. The essential fatty acids and vitamins in rosehip oil are readily absorbed by the skin. With its neutral pH balance and anti-inflammatory properties, rosehip oil keeps skin balanced and healthy, helping to protect against cell degeneration caused by bacteria and oxidants.

jojoba oil *Simmondsia chinensis*; **heavyweight**

Jojoba oil is the liquid that comes from the seed of the jojoba plant, which is a shrub native to southern Arizona, southern California, and northwestern Mexico. Although called an oil, it is actually a liquid plant wax, meaning its chemical structure differs from that of other vegetable oils.

Jojoba has been used in folk medicine for many ailments. Today, jojoba is especially useful for protecting and soothing the skin and is used to treat acne, psoriasis, sunburn, and chapped skin.

Our sebaceous glands are microscopic glands in our skin that secrete an oily or waxy matter called sebum. The texture and benefits of sebum are very similar to those of jojoba oil. As we age, our sebaceous glands produce less sebum, which is why we get dry skin and hair. Jojoba oil can play the role of sebum, moisturizing our skin and hair when our body stops doing it naturally.

borage oil *Borago officinalis;* **heavyweight**

Borage oil comes from the seeds of the borage plant, sometimes known as starflower.

Borage oil is a strong anti-inflammatory because it contains one of the highest levels of the fatty acid known as GLA—gamma-linolenic acid. GLA is one type of omega-6 "essential" fatty acids that the body cannot make on its own, so we must get it from outside sources, such as borage oil. GLA has been shown to correct deficiencies in skin lipids (oils).

When the skin can't produce enough protective oils of its own, the result is increased inflammation and skin flare-ups, so borage oil can help to address these sorts of problems. One of the most well-researched uses for borage oil is treating inflammatory skin disorders such as eczema.

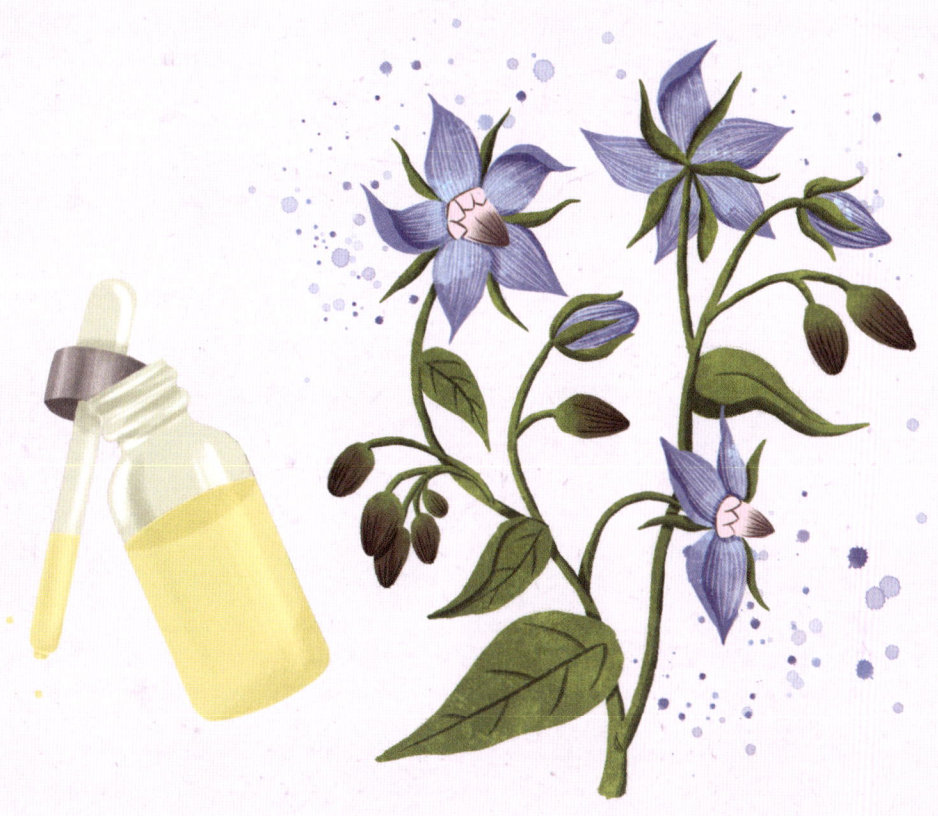

essential oils

Essential oils are remarkably clever. Their capabilities are endless on both physical and mental levels. Each one has its own unique and effective set of properties which, when synergistically combined with other essential oils, make the most powerful remedies believable.

The beautiful fragrances of essential oils are magnified by blending them together. The power of fragrance to transport imagination to memories make essential oils even more spectacular, in that they can affect your physiology on both mental and physical levels, meaning there's a powerhouse of treatments in just a few tiny drops.

how to use essential oils

As you will see over the following pages, there are a huge range of uses for essential oils, but in terms of natural skincare, they are excellent additions to facial oils.

To make a facial oil, add 2 drops in total of essential oil to 1 tablespoon (10 ml) of base oil. Every ingredient is diligently weighed and measured for commercial products, but when you are making them for yourself, this is the perfect dilution. It is worth buying some 0.34-fl oz (10-ml) bottles for your blends, as this will allow for greater precision. For recipes for some of my favorite blends, see pages 96–97.

precautions

Essential oils need to be used with care. Never use them neat (without dilution) as they are extremely concentrated, with the exception of lavender and tea tree which are just as concentrated but can be used neat occasionally (see pages 85 and 86).

Use essential oils as directed by the supplier and don't be tempted to use more than recommended. Since they smell so

recipes for super skin

lovely, you might be tempted to add a few more drops, but this can cause problems such as tingly skin, headaches, and nausea.

If you are pregnant, have a medical condition, or are on medication, take advice from a professional aromatherapist. Most essential oils used correctly will be fine, but it is better and important to be informed. (People get very concerned about the safety of essential oils without realizing that they are used prolifically in the flavor industry and that they may be glugging them down with their fizzy drinks!)

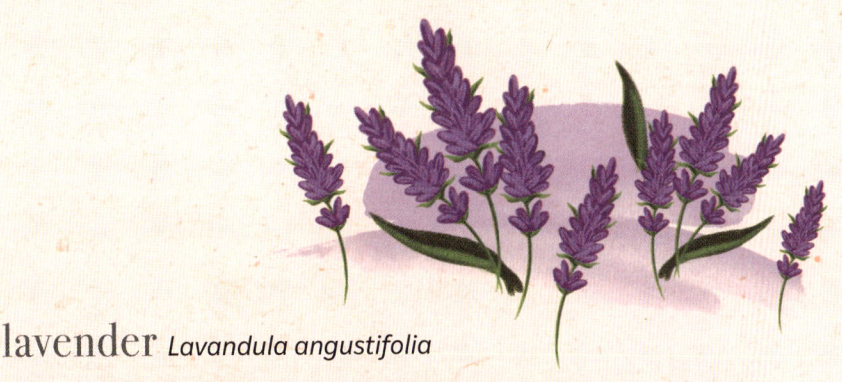

lavender *Lavandula angustifolia*

Ancient texts tell us that lavender essential oil has been used for medicinal and religious purposes for over 2,500 years. The Romans used it for bathing, cooking, and scenting the air. Today, lavender is the most used essential oil in the world.

The word lavender comes from the Latin *lavare* which means "to wash." As the name suggests, it is the most beautiful cleansing oil available, and not only does it cleanse the skin but it also has a cleansing effect on the mind—its fragrance is so calming that it provides a sense of clarity and a fresh start.

In skincare: Lavender essential oil is a synergistic oil, which means it blends seamlessly with other oils while also boosting their properties. You can also use it individually—one neat drop of lavender essential oil can be applied to soothe spots, cuts, burns, and bites.

tea tree *Melaleuca alternifolia*

Tea tree, sometimes known as ti tree, is one of the most extensively researched and provenly effective essential oils. It has a long history of use by the Aboriginal people of Australia where it grows prolifically.

During the Second World War, tea tree essential oil was a general issue in Australian soldiers' backpacks as it has such wide and varied medicinal uses. It is unusual in that it is effective against all three infectious categories—bacteria, fungi, and viruses. It is a powerful immunostimulant, encouraging the body's immune system to fight any of these organisms with great effect. Tea tree is also perfect for cold and flu blends when combined with oils such as eucalyptus and peppermint and diluted in a base oil.

In skincare: Tea tree essential oil can be used sparingly in neat form on spots, cuts, and stings and at the first sign of cold sores. In oil blends and washes, tea tree is good for oily and troublesome skin types.

TEA TREE HEALING

Tea tree essential oil can be used with lemon essential oil to treat warts and verrucas. Apply one neat drop of tea tree oil to the area, immediately covering with a plaster after each application. Repeat daily, alternating between tea tree and lemon oil. After about a week, the wart or verruca should start to dry out, at which point continue applying the oils on alternate days but without covering with a plaster anymore. Parts of the wart or verruca will start to drop off. Fight the urge to "pick" the bits off or you might cause bleeding, which will take you back to the beginning! The area might end up a little dry, so rub in some jojoba oil to re-nourish the skin.

chamomile *Anthemis nobilis*

Chamomile is one of the most ancient medicinal herbs known to mankind. Many different preparations of chamomile have been developed over the years, and the most popular is in the form of herbal tea, with more than 1 million cups consumed per day! But many people don't know that chamomile essential oil is even more effective than the tea.

Chamomile essential oil can help relieve skin irritations that may be due to food allergies or sensitivities. It is a natural mood booster and can help reduce feelings of depression. Its relaxant properties make it a valuable remedy for PMS symptoms, and it can even help clear up acne that may appear because of hormonal fluctuations. Its relaxing properties can also help promote healthy sleep and fight insomnia.

In skincare: Chamomile promotes smooth, healthy skin and relieves irritations because of its anti-inflammatory and antibacterial properties. It can be used blended with a carrier oil or balm as a natural remedy for eczema, wounds, ulcers, gout, skin irritations, bruises, burns, cracked nipples (wash off before breastfeeding), chicken pox, ear infections, poison ivy rash, and nappy rash.

rose geranium *Pelargonium graveolens*

Rose geranium essential oil is extracted through the steam distillation of the stems and leaves of the rose geranium plant. This beautiful oil can also alleviate anxiety, lessen fatigue, and promote emotional wellness by balancing hormones, which in turn uplifts your mood. It is also used as a natural insect repellent.

In skincare: Applied by the ancient Egyptians to promote beautiful and radiant skin, rose geranium essential oil is now used to treat acne and reduce inflammation. It also has the power to minimize the look of wrinkles because it tightens facial skin and slows down the effects of aging by promoting new cell growth.

essential oils

bergamot *Citrus aurantium bergamia*

Bergamot essential oil comes from the rind of the bergamot citrus fruit which is a cross between an orange and a lemon. It is extracted through cold compression, as opposed to the steam distillation of many other essential oils.

Bergamot is an antidepressant and a stimulating essential oil, creating a feeling of freshness, joy, and energy. Flavonoids, which are present in bergamot oil, are relaxants. They soothe nerves and reduce nervous tension, anxiety, and stress, which in turn can help with problems such as sleeplessness, high blood pressure, insomnia, and depression.

In skincare: Bergamot essential oil can help with scarring, pigmentation, and other marks on the skin.

grapefruit *Citrus paradisi*

Grapefruit essential oil comes from the peel of the fruit of the citrus paradisi grapefruit tree. As one of the most versatile essential oils, the aroma of grapefruit oil is clean, fresh, and a little bit bitter, just like the fruit itself.

Grapefruit oil is naturally high in antioxidants and phytochemicals that reduce oxidative stress and disease-causing inflammation. Many of the benefits of grapefruit essential oil are due to one of its main constituents, limonene (which makes up about 88 percent to 95 percent of the oil). In addition to limonene, grapefruit essential oil contains other powerful antioxidants, including vitamin C, myrcene, terpinene, pinene, and citronellol.

In skincare: Grapefruit essential oil is a great addition to cleansers (one drop in 1 fl oz (30 ml) of fractionated coconut oil works well) and blends for oily skin. It has antibacterial and anti-inflammatory properties, making it effective for spot-prone skin.

mandarin *Citrus nobilis*

Mandarin essential oil comes from the outer rind of the fruit. The oil is extracted through a cold-pressing process. With a history dating back thousands of years to traditional Chinese medicine, mandarin is known to be the sweetest and most calming of all citrus essential oils. In France, it is known as "the children oil" because it is so gentle.

Mandarin can help ward against infection of irritated skin by preventing bacterial and fungal development.

In skincare: Mandarin essential oil is useful in helping to reduce acne and oily skin, brighten skin tone, diminish the appearance of scars and age spots, and improve wrinkles by minimizing the effects of stress.

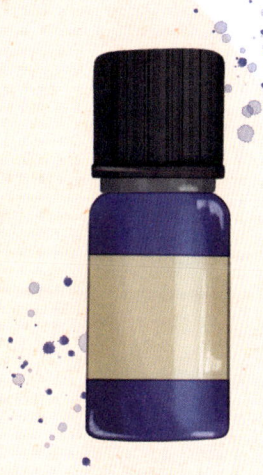

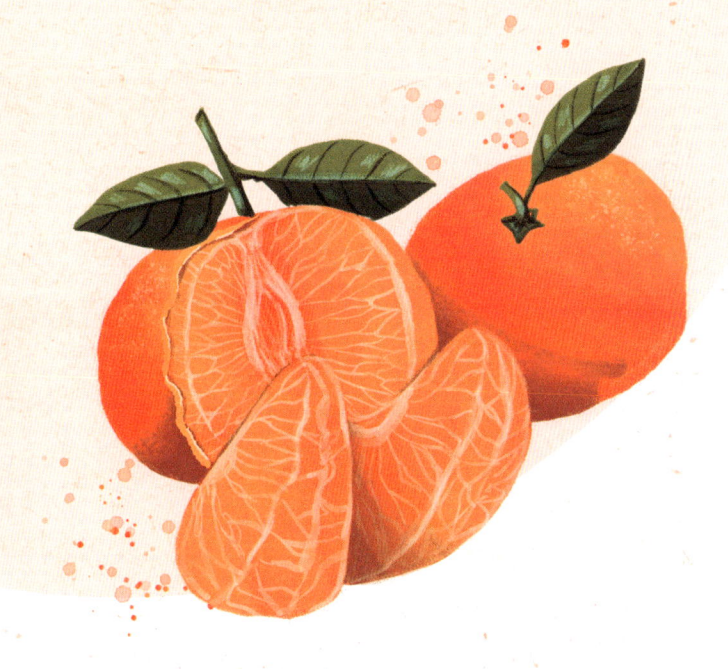

sandalwood *Santalum spicata*

Sandalwood essential oil comes from the wood of the sandalwood tree and is one of the most expensive woods in the world. The oil used to come mainly from the Indian *Santalum album* tree, but it became so exploited that India stopped the free use of the slow-growing trees for essential oil extraction and furniture making. Lots of furniture was traditionally made from sandalwood as it was renowned for keeping ants at bay—a clear indication of what a good insect repellent it is.

I now use Australian sandalwood essential oil (*santalum spicata*), which has an almost identical fragrance and the same wonderful therapeutic properties as the Indian oil, but it is sustainably harvested.

Sandalwood has always been used in perfumes, home fragrances, and skincare, but over the past few years it has become very popular in high-end fragrances and even laundry products. Its fragrance is sensuous and grounding, giving a real sense of calm. As a summer fragrance, it is pure golden sunlight; in winter, a warm blanket.

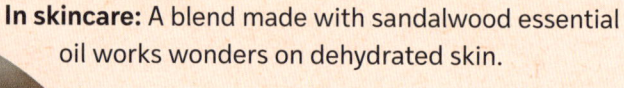

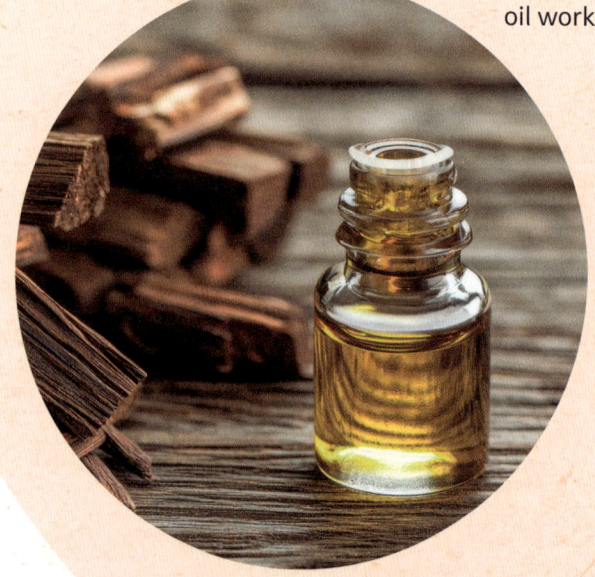

In skincare: A blend made with sandalwood essential oil works wonders on dehydrated skin.

frankincense *Boswellia carterii*

Frankincense essential oil comes from the resin of certain types of *Boswellia* tree. The word frankincense comes from the term *franc encens*, which means "quality incense" in old French.

It is believed that the oil transmits messages to the limbic system of the brain, which influences the nervous system. When inhaled, it has been shown to reduce heart rate and slow down breathing, which is said to put you in a trance-like state—for this reason it is used in churches as incense.

Frankincense essential oil can also help reduce symptoms associated with menstruation and menopause by balancing hormone levels and can ease anxiety and depression.

In skincare: This oil has the ability to strengthen skin and improve its tone and elasticity, helping to prevent wrinkles and naturally slow down signs of aging. It can also be used to help reduce acne blemishes and the appearance of large pores, is useful for fading stretch marks, surgery scars, and marks associated with pregnancy, and is great for healing dry or cracked skin.

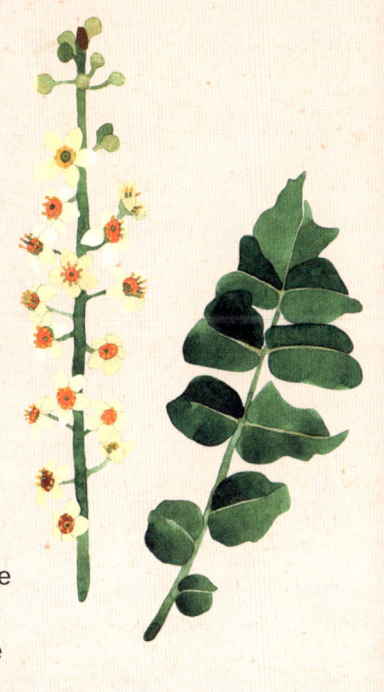

cedarwood *Cedrus atlantica*

Cedarwood essential oil is extracted through steam distillation from wood pieces of the cedar tree. Cedars are the trees mentioned most in the Bible. They are regarded as a symbol of protection, wisdom, and abundance.

Cedarwood essential oil improves focus and wisdom: it is also comforting, soothing, and reassuring with a warm, woody tone. It is known to bring people together and improve personal outlook and self-esteem, as well as being said to have the ability to change a person's perspective!

In skincare: With its anti-inflammatory properties, cedarwood essential oil can help reduce skin irritations and fungal infections, repel bugs, stimulate metabolism, cleanse toxins, and fight acne. Since the oil is an astringent, it tightens loose muscles and skin and creates a feeling of firmness and youth.

essential oils

what are hydrosols?

Hydrosols (also known as hydrolats) are a lovely addition to natural skincare and you can even use them as a subtle natural perfume.

Hydrosols are a by-product of the extraction process of essential oils. There was a time when hydrosols were thrown away, but now money and effort have been invested in keeping the precious liquids clean and safe for use. When an essential oil is extracted from a plant using a distillation still, water is boiled so that steam rises through the plant matter to release the aromatic oil. The oil separates and floats to the top as the steam condenses. The oil can then be removed, and the remaining water is called a hydrosol. This water contains all the beneficial essence of the plant, but in much smaller amounts.

    Hydrosols should not be confused with flower waters. They are, of course, flower waters, but they can also be fruit, herb, or even resin waters. Also, some flower waters are a combination of fragrance, water, solubilizers, and preservatives. Real hydrosols do not need preservatives because they have so much residue essential oil in them that they self-preserve. Some companies use a preservative in their hydrosol to prolong its shelf life, but I search for 100 percent natural, organic hydrosols and they are simply divine. I also find them quite robust in terms of their shelf life, as long as they are kept out of direct sunlight and in a cool place.

    There are myriad hydrosols. Rose and neroli or orange blossom are well known, but there are many more choices, and just like essential oils, they each have their own therapeutic properties. In fact, some people call the therapeutic use of hydrosols the new aromatherapy. They are so useful because they require very few precautions and, like essential oils, they can be combined with one another to make different natural remedies.

how to use hydrosols

For natural skincare, hydrosols make wonderful cleansers, toners, and facial spritzes. My personal favorite use for them is to spritz my face and neck with a hydrosol before applying facial oil, as this allows the oil to distribute beautifully.

If you have only ever used cream or lotion on your face and neck and are cautious of using oil, here is something to consider. Creams and lotions are made up of oils and/or waxes and water. For these two elements to combine, they need an emulsifier, and because of the water content they also need preservatives. If you apply a hydrosol before your facial oil, you effectively have a cream without any of the added chemicals. Apply the oil to your damp skin. It feels wonderful and everything is absorbed quickly and easily, with no oily residue whatsoever. Give it a try!

A hydrosol can be diluted with distilled water, but definitely does not need to be unless you want it to go further—but then you run the risk of contaminating the hydrosol and making it go off sooner than it might otherwise (see page 94).

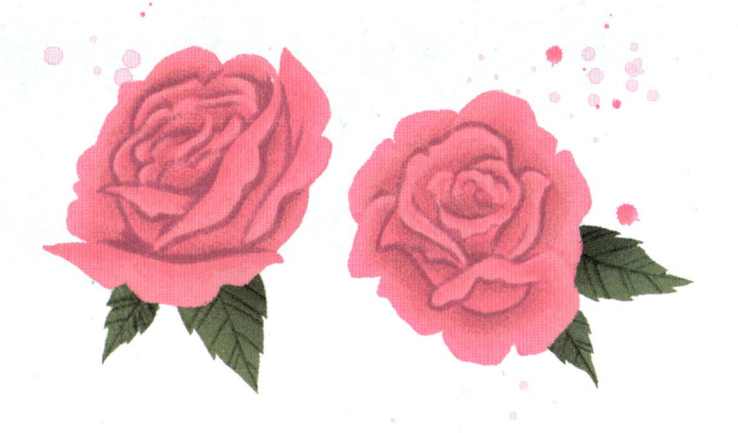

choosing and storing oils

All natural products need to be carefully stored. If they are natural, they should not have any preservatives in them, so they rely on your careful handling to last their full shelf life. Always read the ingredients list to check that they really are natural.

storage

Natural products are heat- and light-sensitive. The most effective way to store oils is in dark glass bottles, which is how essential oils are usually sold (or the bottle has a protective outer layer), but base oils sometimes come in clear glass bottles. If this is the case, make sure to keep them in a cupboard away from heat and light. Natural products must also be kept airtight, and you should avoid putting your fingers in them or around the lids as your fingers can carry germs and moisture.

Base oils and hydrosols have the shortest shelf lives, which can be anything from six months to two years depending on the way they are handled and stored. Base oils can easily become rancid (if they are turning rancid they start to crystallize around the neck of the bottle, change color, and smell like old walnuts) and hydrosols smell rank when they are off, a bit like wet rags that have been left damp for too long.

Essential oils, when stored and handled correctly, can last far longer than it says on the label. Some essential oils have been found intact in pyramids! These will undoubtably have been resinous oils, such as frankincense, sandalwood, and cedarwood. Citrus oils, on the other hand, lose their fragrance within a year or so, and even quicker if not stored correctly. The best indication of whether an essential oil is still good for use is its fragrance. If it does not smell good, it should not be used. If it is a dull brownish color, this also means it has gone off.

quality

If possible, it is worth using organic oils. Organic essential oils in particular have more clarity of fragrance. Whether you buy organic or non-organic, there are a few things to look out for.

Always look carefully at the labeling. The Latin name of the plant that the oil has been extracted from should always be stated. This is because there are different strains of plants that oil can be extracted from, and one can differ quite dramatically from another both therapeutically and fragrance-wise. If the ingredients label states more than the Latin name and includes water/aqua and other chemicals, be aware that this will not be a pure essential oil or base oil.

For essential oils, the word "pure" should also appear on the label. A few oils are "absolutes" or "resins" instead, and this is fine—it indicates the extraction method. (The word "pure" does not appear on absolutes and resins.) Read up on what you are buying; most good suppliers give lots of information on their website.

Prices of essential oils vary widely. This is because the yield of essential oil from each plant type is different. Orange essential oil is prolific, whereas roses only yield a tiny amount of oil. Some oils, such as sandalwood, take years to become harvestable. Therefore, when you see that one essential oil costs much more than another, there is probably a good reason for it.

Don't go out and buy lots of oils. Buy a few, or even just one or two, and test them for fragrance, texture, and compatibility with your skin. Read suppliers' advice about the suitability of specific oils. Good suppliers will have product support on their website or packaging. Gather information and refine your choices as you go, as there is a lot to learn. Stick to pure essential oils and cold-pressed carrier oils to begin with.

facial oil recipes

These blends will leave your skin bright, nourished, and happy and are perfect to use before facial yoga, facial reflexology, gua sha, or cryotherapy.

A 0.34-fl oz (10-ml) bottle of face oil is enough for approximately one week's worth of usage when applied once per day. To clean the bottle when it is empty, simply wash in hot, soapy water and make sure it is completely dry before refilling it. The bottles do not have to be sterilized, as they are for small amounts and don't need to last for ages. Plus, the essential oils themselves will combat any potential germs. The best bottles to use are made of dark-colored glass, or you can store clear bottles in a cabinet or refrigerator.

Facial oils work better on damp skin, so spray a little hydrosol or damp a flannel in a bowl of warm water and dab it over your face and neck before applying your face oil.

For each of the following blends, pour all the oils into a small, clean, screw-top bottle and shake to mix. Shake before each use.

revitalizing morning facial oil

This recipe is great for all skin types and will "wake up" your face, no matter how tired you are feeling.

1 tablespoon (10 ml) peach kernel oil

1 drop of mandarin essential oil

1 drop of grapefruit essential oil

balancing facial oil

This recipe will address both oily and dry patches, leaving your skin with a more even texture.

1 teaspoon (5 ml) peach kernel oil

1 teaspoon (5 ml) argan oil

1 drop of rose geranium essential oil

1 drop of lavender essential oil

nighttime nourishing facial oil

This wonderfully rich and luxurious oil will "feed" undernourished, parched skin.

1 tablespoon (10 ml) jojoba oil
1 drop of frankincense essential oil
1 drop of sandalwood essential oil

sensitive skin facial oil

Made with the gentlest of oils, this blend will soothe and protect even the most delicate skin.

1 tablespoon (10 ml) calendula oil
1 drop of chamomile essential oil
1 drop of lavender essential oil

FACIAL SERUMS

What is a facial serum, and how does it differ from a facial oil? In truth, the two terms are interchangeable, and some makers of facial serums feel strongly that a facial serum should contain water and other added ingredients such as hyaluronic acid, retinol, and vitamin C—but for those wanting truly natural facial skincare (as discussed on page 74), water in a product requires unnatural additions, such as emulsifiers and preservatives. Having worked in natural skincare for decades, I would personally consider a natural facial serum to be a blend of oils more targeted to the needs of specific skin conditions than a regular facial oil. Of course, certain makers of face oils will describe them in this way, meaning it comes down to marketing.

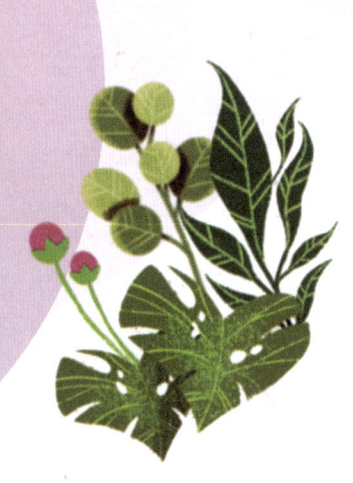

98 recipes for super skin

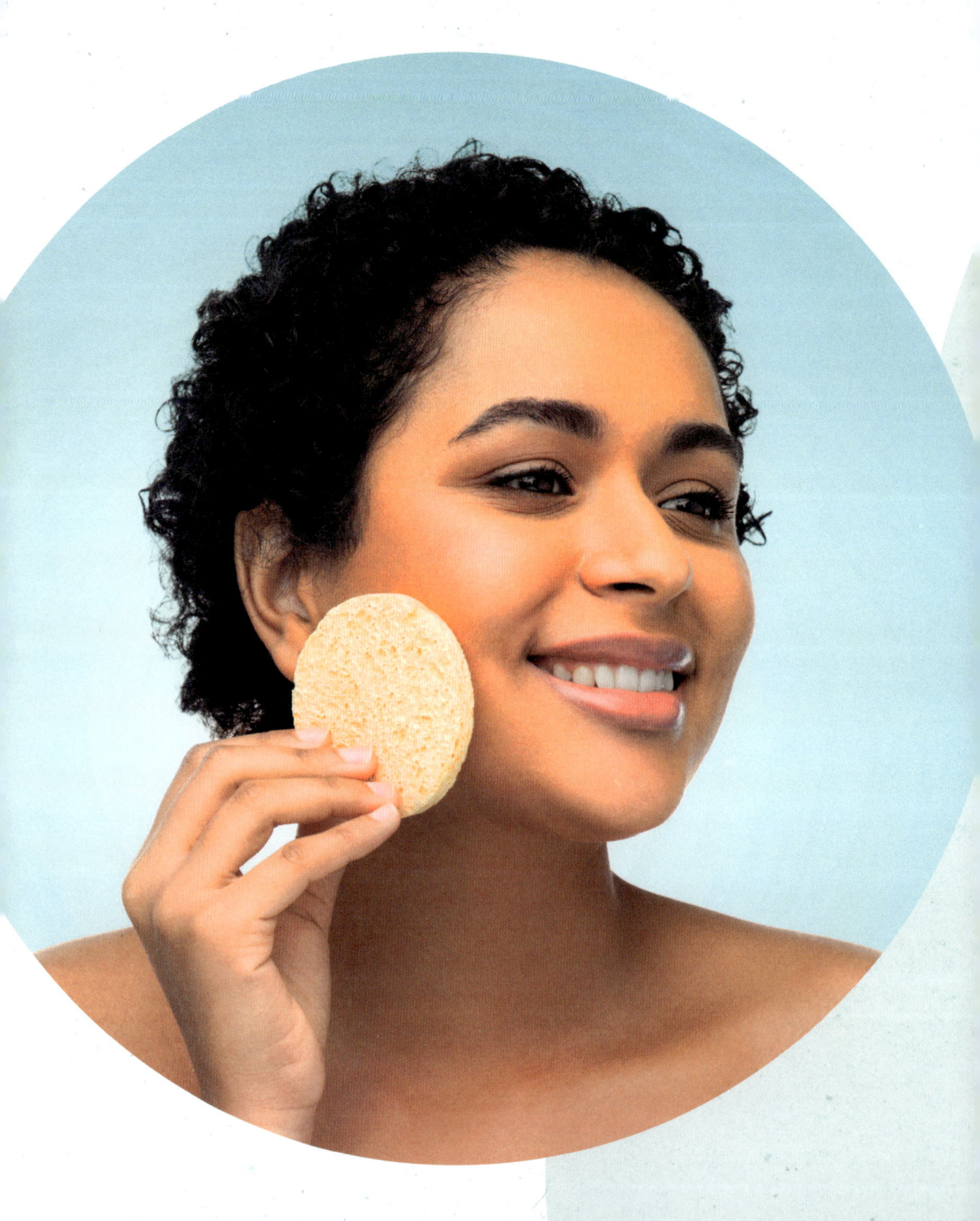

exfoliation

Our skin sheds skin cells at a rate of about 600,000 per day! If we don't get rid of them, they can hang around, making our skin look dull and congested.

Luckily, exfoliation is easier than you think. Your exfoliant doesn't have to be very coarse or rough. There are simple, natural ways to exfoliate without stripping your skin of its natural flora, and these can be incorporated into your skincare routine.

- Use a slightly rough flannel or reusable cleansing pad when washing or drying your face.
- Make an exfoliator by grinding up dried aduki beans. (You could use dry rice, dried flowers, or dried herbs instead, if you wish.) Apply this to damp skin with a gentle, circular massage. Less is more. You don't need to scrub your face red to get it to glow. Rinse off to finish.
- A face steam can help to exfoliate your skin. Add 10 drops of an essential oil such as lavender or tea tree (or you can combine the two essential oils—5 drops of each) to a bowl filled with around 4¼ cups (1 liter) of hot but not boiling water, then hold your face over the bowl with a towel over your head for 5 minutes. To finish, dry your face with a clean hand towel, rubbing gently as you do so. Do this once a week.

CHAPTER 5

natural wellness

With all the exercises, treatments, products, and potions in the world, it is hard to have a natural glow if you don't feel good. This chapter looks at a variety of ways to improve your health and well-being, both physically and mentally, which will in turn be reflected in your face.

the vagus nerve

Most research into the vagus nerve has only been done over the last 20 years. Having an understanding of how it works can be very useful in helping us have control over our ability to cope with stressful situations and our general sense of well-being, which in turn can give us a natural glow.

There are 12 paired sets of cranial nerves, which stem from the brain and they affect all our senses: taste, smell, sight, hearing, and touch. The cranial nerves serve our parasympathetic nervous system, sometimes called the "rest and digest" nervous system, which can relax us and make us calmer. (Our sympathetic nervous system is the system that is responsible for our "fight or flight" response to stress.)

The vagus nerve is the longest and largest pair of cranial nerves, stretching from our brain to our intestines, affecting all our organs along the way. The Latin word *vagus* means "wandering," which is appropriate as it journeys throughout the body. In effect, it is a highway for neurotransmitters from the gut to the brain, affecting sleep, mood, stress levels, and hunger. These neurotransmitters go both ways—from the brain to the body and vice versa—but 80 percent of information comes from the body to the brain and only 20 percent from the brain to the body.

This artwork shows how the vagus nerve is linked to all our organs—including the lungs, heart, liver, stomach, and intestines. (This is a simplified diagram: in reality the nerve descends from the brain as a pair of nerves and branches out throughout the body.)

102 natural wellness

So, what does this mean? As I'm sure you all know from experience, sadness and stress can cause stomach upset, but your stomach upset can also cause sadness and stress. Serotonin, which is a natural mood boosting hormone, is 90 percent produced in the gut, so if you have a happy gut, you have a good chance of feeling happy, and this happiness will show in your face.

Toning our vagus nerve with some simple exercises and activities can give us greater control over our well-being, mood, stress levels, and ability to focus.

vagus nerve exercise

Below is a well-established exercise by Stanley Rosenburg, author of *The Healing Power of the Vagus Nerve*. It can be done quickly and easily by anyone, and it works best if you do it two or three times a day. To begin with, practice it lying down, but once you are comfortable with the sensation of exercising your eyes and soothing your vagus nerve in this way, you can do it sitting up straight.

1 Lace the fingers of both hands together and cradle them behind your head, so you can feel the bones of your skull in the palms of your hands. Take a few deep breaths.

2 Look to the right without moving your head. Stay in this position for about a minute or until you feel the need to sigh, yawn, or take a deep breath, which signals that you are starting to relax. The feeling may not come the first time you do this exercise, but it will in time.

3 Slowly bring your eyes back to the center and rest for a few seconds, then repeat on the other side.

4 You only need to do this once on each side. You will feel calm and relaxed, and your neck may feel freer, too.

connecting the dots

LI-20 is an acupuncture pressure point that can stimulate the large intestines. As explained earlier, messages travel from the stomach and intestines to the brain via the vagus nerve, so by stimulating this pressure point we can send calming, happy signals to our brain. This point is widely used in Thai and Japanese massage and in Traditional Chinese Medicine. In Thai massage it is called Golden Bamboo, and in Traditional Chinese Medicine its name is Welcoming Fragrance.

Stimulating this point improves the circulation of blood to the face, makes the face more responsive to social interaction, and can open the nostrils to improve breathing, which is very useful when you are congested or suffering from hayfever.

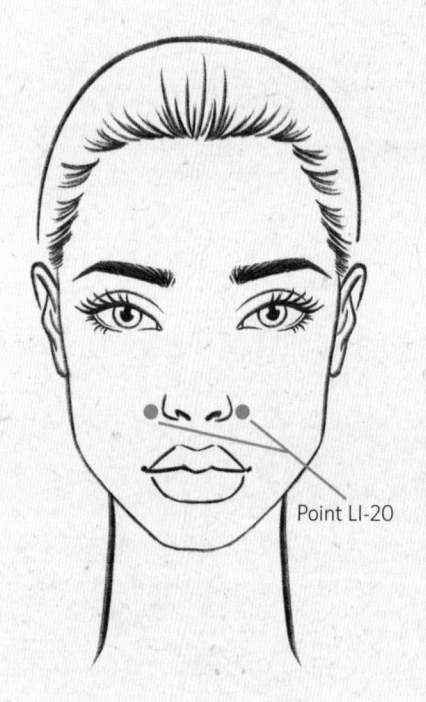

Point LI-20

1 Sit at a table or desk, making sure you are sitting up straight and can breathe freely, and rest your elbows on the surface.

2 Locate LI-20 with your index fingers—a little way out from the little dents at the base of your nose, under your cheekbones. It is often a little tender here. Gently press LI-20 with your index fingers and allow the weight of your head to push down a little for a few seconds, then release the pressure. Repeat three times.

3 Press LI-20 again, but stay in this position for a few minutes longer this time. You will start to feel the bone under the muscles of your face. Allow your fingers to move up and down by gently rocking your head forward and back. Don't push too hard or for too long. It should feel like a pleasant ache.

4 Take your fingers away and relax. When you have finished, you might find that your face has been stimulated in such a way that you want to smile. This is a pathway for social engagement, which is another way to stimulate our vagus nerve (see opposite).

natural wellness

toning your vagus nerve

Sometimes, a face can "set" in a scowl or frown, making it almost impossible to have a natural glow, but a toned vagus nerve can give us a sense of well-being that literally shows in our faces. There are many quick and easy ways to tone your vagus nerve, so you have some control over how you feel and how you react in stressful situations. Just about anything that relaxes, soothes, or happily distracts you will contribute to vagus nerve stimulation. Here are a few:

- Humming
- Gargling
- Singing
- Chanting
- Cold water—splash your face with cold water, then hold your breath for 10 seconds (see page 108)
- Grounding—walk with bare feet, even for just a few minutes
- Meditating (see page 116)
- Head and neck massage
- Social engagement (see below)—especially being with people you love

PEOPLE POWER

Social engagement—that is, interacting with other people—is one of the best ways to tone our vagus nerve. All 12 cranial nerves are involved in social interaction. When we look at someone, we naturally mirror them, utilizing myriad facial nerves and muscles. The more we interact with others, the more empathetic we become, and the more toned our faces and vagus nerve become.

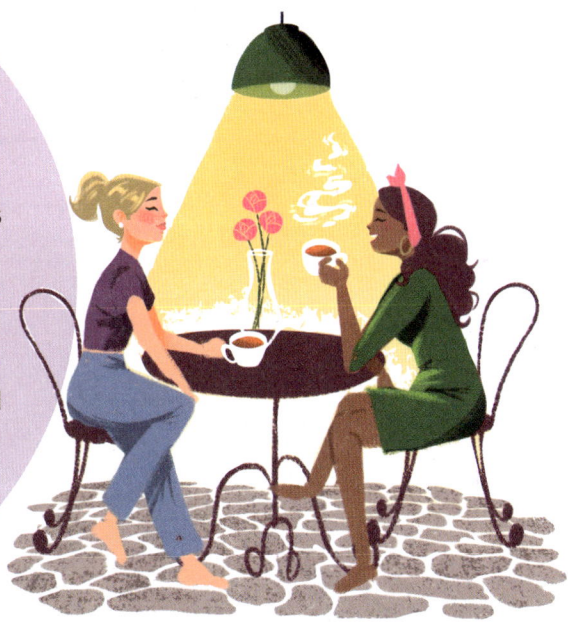

the chakras

The chakras are an ancient Hindu and Buddhist system that links the body and spirit with energy centers that run down the middle of the body.

Meditating on your chakras or having a Reiki practitioner work on them can be a wonderfully therapeutic experience. Just being familiar with them is also a very useful tool. (The chakras are also linked to facial reflexology points—see page 41.)

chakra associations

There are seven main chakras, and each one can have an effect on you physically, spiritually, and mentally.

- The Crown chakra relates to feeling enlightened and spiritual.
- The Third Eye chakra relates to feeling intuitive and imaginative.
- The Throat chakra relates to feeling confident and focused.
- The Heart chakra relates to feeling love and compassion.
- The Solar Plexus chakra relates to feeling confident and balanced.
- The Sacral chakra relates to feeling creative and sensual.
- The Root chakra relates to feeling grounded and secure.

chakra meditation

If one of your chakras is blocked, energy in the corresponding areas will be flagging. If this concept resonates with you and you have a feeling of stagnancy in any specific chakra area, try meditating on the corresponding chakra as follows:

Take your thoughts to the chakra you feel needs some work. Breathe in and out slowly and deeply, while imagining this chakra as a ball of light that expands when you breathe in and gets smaller when you breathe out.

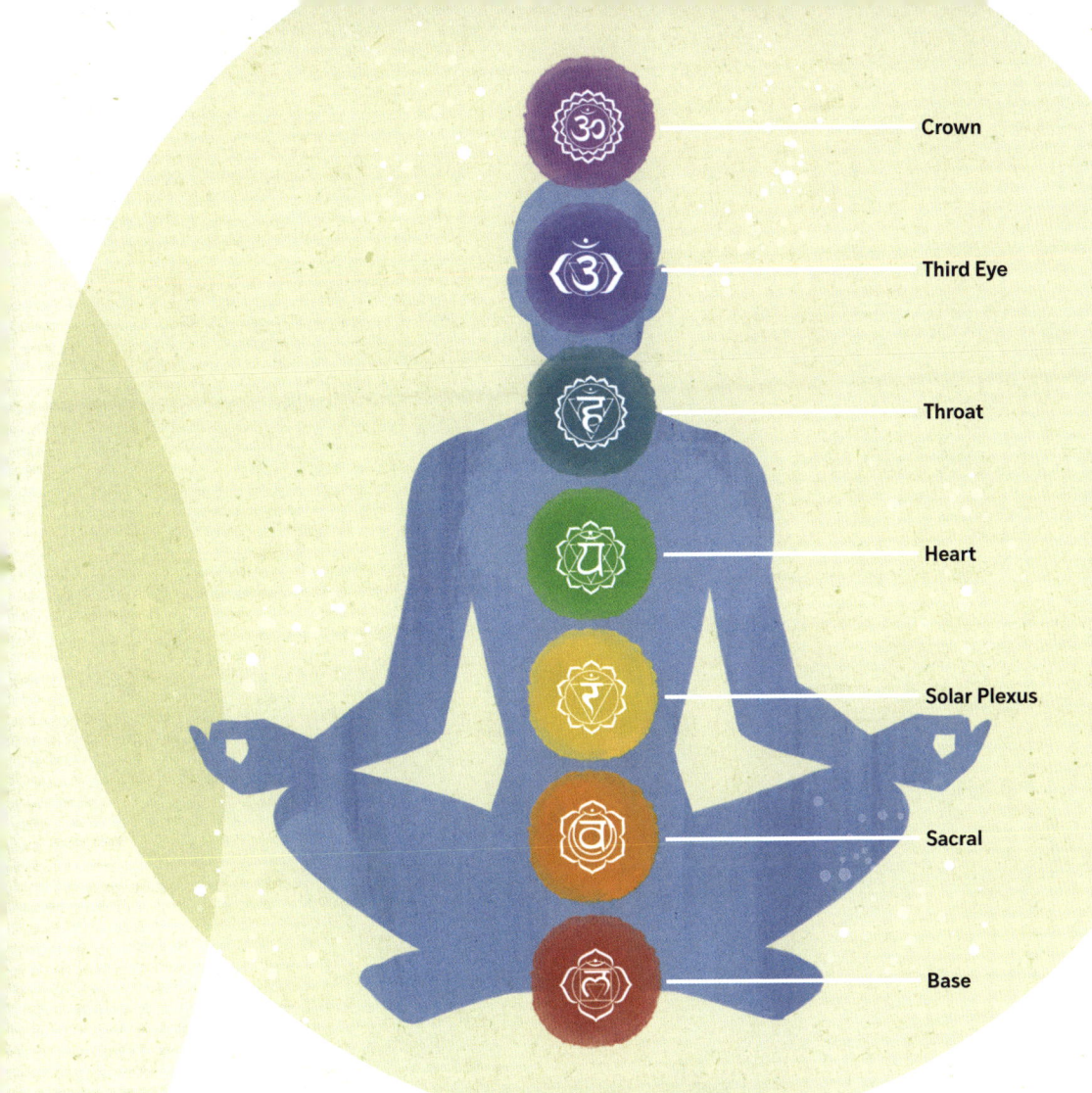

- Crown
- Third Eye
- Throat
- Heart
- Solar Plexus
- Sacral
- Base

Think of the feeling this chakra relates to (see list opposite). If you want to feel confident and focused, for instance, think of a beautiful ball of blue light that is filling you with calmness and strength via the area of your Throat chakra. Think of calm, flow, clarity, and openness. Stay with this feeling for 10 slow breaths.

Now cast your mind over each of the other chakras and imagine them all joined by a beautiful thread of silver light, balancing your body and spirit. Take another 10 slow breaths, imagining pure energy running up and down this silver thread.

the chakras

cold water therapy

If you are seeking a natural glow, look no further than cold water therapy, which is like a reboot for the body.

Water therapy, also known as hydrotherapy, can be in a bath, shower, the sea, a river, swimming pool, jacuzzi, or sauna—anywhere you can immerse yourself in water for a therapeutic or relaxing effect. Types of water therapy include:

- Exercising in water for low impact, so that strain is placed on the joints.
- Soaking in a warm bath with mineral salts and/or essential oils to ease muscle pain and relax your mind and body.
- Swimming in the sea or a pool.
- Taking a shower to wash away stress.
- Soaking your feet in cool water on a hot day.

However, the best option for a radiant effect is cold water therapy—exposing yourself to water as cold as you can bear. When your body is suddenly subjected to cold, the surface blood in your capillaries (the tiny blood vessels on the surface of your skin) is pushed to the core of your body, giving your heart and brain an influx of blood, which is wonderfully invigorating. Your skin will appear temporarily pale, but will quickly become naturally glowing once the blood vessels dilate again as your body warms up.

After cold water therapy, your body feels instantly more awake, tingly, and raring to go. Your mind feels more alert, and suddenly all those boulders that were in your way disappear. Research into cold water therapy suggests it has the ability to improve mental health and depression and to reduce anxiety.

It is not for the fainthearted, but there are degrees of cold water therapy, and you can start slowly and carefully, then build up to colder water and a longer time in the cold water. Why would I, you might well ask? Well, apart from the reasons mentioned above, it becomes addictive. Once you have mastered the art of simply turning your shower to cold, you will be pulled not pushed into doing it, because you won't want to miss the fantastic feeling and glow that it instantly gives you.

practicing cold water therapy

It is simple to incorporate this type of hydrotherapy into your daily routine. If you want a quick wakeup fix that will give your skin a lovely glow, you can simply splash your face with icy cold water. Not only will this wake you up, but the vasodilation (widening of your blood vessels) that it promotes is like a mini workout for your complexion and will tighten up your skin.

For a whole body experience, shower as normal with the water at your regular temperature. You can slowly make the water colder until it feels almost freezing, and keep it at that temperature for up to three minutes. Alternatively, and I feel this is the better way, once you have washed and are ready to get out of your shower, switch the water to cold and stay underneath for up to three minutes. If you have a hand-held shower, make sure to cover all areas of your body, especially those parts that might have injuries. Cold water speeds up the rate of recovery of injuries by reducing pain and swelling, and is satisfyingly numbing.

Ice-cold plunge pools are the ultimate in cold water therapy, but personally I have yet to pluck up the courage! At home, why not try immersing yourself in a warm bath first, then taking a cold shower before you get out?

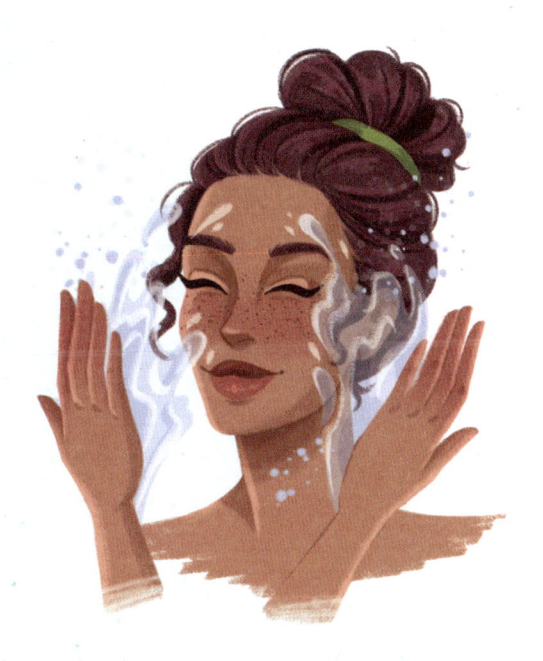

CAUTION

A word of warning: If you have heart problems, high blood pressure, or deep vein thrombosis, or if you suffer from epilepsy, consult a doctor or health professional before trying cold water therapy. Cold water therapy is not suitable for pregnant women.

breathwork

Good breathing is intrinsic to good health. Every cell in the body needs oxygen, and when we breathe in, our bloodstream takes up that oxygen and delivers it to all those cells. This is why it is so important to breathe well.

Of course, many of the techniques we have covered in earlier chapters will promote good breathing. The synergy between all the practices I have shared so far is strong. Even if you have a condition that makes your breathing less than optimal, you can strengthen and improve your breathing using breathwork. Breathing exercises can build your lung capacity, and improve your circulation, mood, concentration, and energy levels. These exercises engage your parasympathetic nervous system, which calms and relaxes you by overriding your sympathetic nervous system (the nerves in charge of your "fight or flight" response to stress). When you are anxious, your breathing becomes short and jagged, which leads to less oxygen going to your brain and results in confusion and panic. Breathwork can counteract this by increasing the amount of oxygen being circulated around your whole body, leaving you with more energy and clarity of thought.

When you breathe normally, your inhalation and exhalation will be fairly even. In breathwork exercises, we control our breath using imaginary patterns to extend, hold, and direct our breath. We want the breath to be smooth and rhythmical, which gives a wonderful feeling of calm. When we extend the out-breath, we become more relaxed. Holding the breath when the lungs are either full or empty (see Box Breath, page 113) focuses the mind and can help put you into a calm and meditative state.

tips for breathwork

The best way to do your breathing practice is sitting upright with your back straight. You can sit on the floor or on a chair. If you are sitting on the floor, cross-legged, half-lotus (cross-legged with one foot on the opposite thigh, the other resting on the ground), or full lotus (cross-legged with both feet resting on their opposite thighs), use a pillow to sit on or to support your knees for comfort if needed. You can also lie down on the floor. If lying down causes any discomfort in your back, placing a pillow under your knees can help. It is important not to be distracted by any discomfort caused by the way you are sitting or lying down.

Keep your shoulders and jaw relaxed throughout. Your eyes are best closed, but if you are doing your breathing exercises on a train or bus, it might be easier to keep them open.

Most breathwork is done through the nose, also known as nasal breathing. This gives you more control over your breath, allowing you to adjust the length of each breath more easily. Nasal breathing also warms, moistens, and filters the air before it enters your lungs.

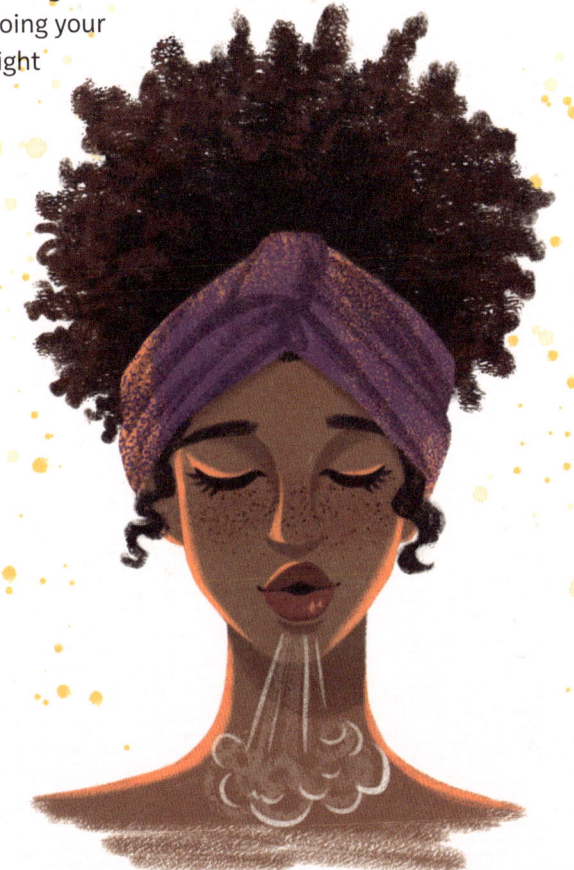

breathwork exercises

There are myriad breathwork exercises, but these are some of my favorites, which are simple to learn.

six breaths per minute

This exercise is also known as coherent breathing. It helps to synchronize your heart rate with your breathing, which helps reduce stress. It involves even breaths in and out through the nose with no holds. The optimum rate of breathing for relaxation is around six breaths per minute. This is the perfect introduction to breathwork. Do this simple exercise anytime and anywhere to quickly create some space in your mind and calm in your body.

1 Breathe in for 5 counts, then breathe out for 5 counts.

2 Repeat ten times.

hand breath

I have always found this simple exercise incredibly useful to send myself back to sleep if I wake in the night, but also to focus my attention quickly when needed. The sensation of gentle touch is supremely relaxing, but this exercise also works well if you just imagine you are tracing the contours of your hand.

1 Hold up your least dominant hand.

2 With the index finger of your other hand, trace the edges of the fingers of the hand you are holding up, starting at the base of your thumb. Breathe in as you trace upward and breathe out as you trace downward. Work your way over every finger until you get to the outside base of your little finger. You can control your breathing by the speed of the finger tracing, which means you can actively slow your breath by slowing down your movement.

3 Work back the other way until you are back at the base of your thumb.

4 Repeat as many times as you like as you fall asleep, or until you feel that your focus has improved.

box breath

This is a very well-known breathing exercise. It is simple to do and good for learning to control your breath. The equal "inhalation, hold, exhalation, hold" sequence is by nature very balancing. Its Sanskrit name *Sama Vritti* means balancing one's mind and body.

1 Picture a box in your mind.

2 Inhale for 4 counts while imagining drawing up the left-hand side of the box.

3 Hold your breath for 4 counts while imagining drawing along the top side of the box.

4 Exhale for 4 counts while imagining drawing down the right-hand side of the box.

5 Hold your breath for 4 counts while imagining drawing the base of the box.

6 Repeat the whole sequence ten times.

cooling breath

I always picture a cartoon frog catching a fly when I do this exercise. In yoga practice it is used to cool the mind and body. It's fantastic on a hot day. Sit upright with your eyes closed for this exercise. You also need to sit rather than lie down, so that you can move your head up and down.

1 Curl your tongue like a straw by sucking the side edges into the center of your tongue inside your mouth. (If you can't curl your tongue, try to make your tongue into a small bowl shape.)

2 Push your rolled tongue through your lips and lift your chin while breathing in air through or over your tongue.

3 Return your head to a straight position and bring your tongue back into your mouth while holding your breath.

4 Lower your chin and breathe out through your nose.

5 Repeat the whole sequence ten times.

breathwork exercises

alternate nostril breathing

This exercise, also known as *Nadi Shodhana*, helps to balance both sides of the brain. The concentration it requires helps calm and clear your mind.

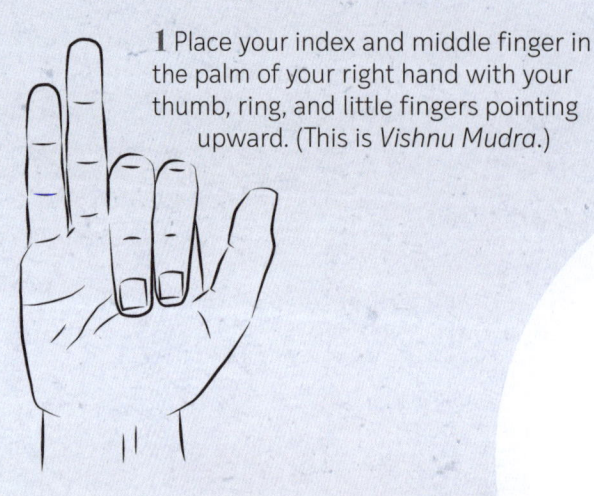

1 Place your index and middle finger in the palm of your right hand with your thumb, ring, and little fingers pointing upward. (This is *Vishnu Mudra*.)

2 Place your thumb over your right nostril to close it, and very lightly place your ring finger on the other nostril, so the air can enter but at a slower rate. Breathe in through the left nostril for 4 counts.

3 Close the left nostril with your ring finger and release the thumb from the right nostril, but keeping the pressure light as you did on the other side. Breathe out through the right nostril for 4 counts.

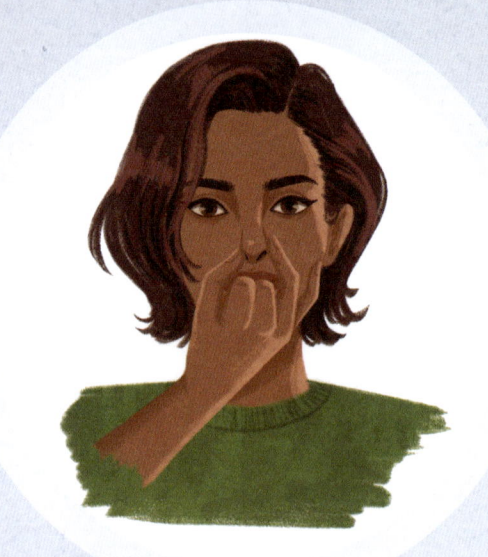

4 Breathe in through the same right nostril for 4 counts, keeping your thumb very lightly over it.

5 Close the right nostril with your thumb and release the ring finger from the left nostril, but keeping the pressure light. Breathe out for 4 counts.

6 Repeat the whole sequence ten times.

natural wellness

extended breath

This exercise increases strength in your lungs and gives you focus. It's about building the length of your breath, which can be quite difficult. If so, keep doing the first couple of rounds to begin with, and try for longer as you get better at it. If you start to feel at all lightheaded, stop and breathe normally and try the exercise another time.

1 Breathe in for 2 counts, pause, breathe out for 4 counts, then pause again.

2 Breathe in for 3 counts, pause, breathe out for 6 counts, then pause once more.

3 Breathe in for 4 counts, pause, breathe out for 8 counts, then pause again.

4 Breathe in for 5 counts, pause, breathe out for 10 counts, then pause again.

5 Breathe in for 6 counts, pause, breathe out for 12 counts, then pause again.

6 Now work the whole sequence in reverse, going from breathing in for 6 counts through to breathing in for 2 counts.

energizing breath

We have talked a lot about using breathwork for relaxation, but this exercise, which involves short exhales while pumping your tummy, can give you energy and leave you refreshed and focused.

1 Breathe in and out a few times, until you feel comfortable.

2 Take a deep breath in and hold for about a second.

3 Exhale through your nose, using short, sharp pumps with your tummy pushing in on each exhale, until all the air is expelled.

4 Repeat ten times.

5 End by taking a few deep breaths in and out.

TRY THIS

By slightly closing off the back of the throat, you can control the rate of inhalation and exhalation more easily. This can make a slight noise within your head which adds to the meditative quality of the Extended Breath exercise.

meditation

Breathwork can also be linked to meditation, which has a positive impact on our sleep, concentration, circulation, and mood. Meditating regularly teaches your brain how to switch off the chatter inside, which is great if you have trouble getting to sleep or getting back to sleep if you wake in the night. You can often feel even more refreshed after meditating than after sleeping.

Simply sit or lie down, and breathe in and out slowly through your nose, letting any thoughts that come into your mind drift away on an imaginary cloud. It might help to count from one to ten repeatedly: Breathe in on one and out on two until you reach ten, then repeat until your mind clears. You could also set yourself a time—even five minutes will do the trick. Build up the amount of time as and when you can. Use an alarm to tell you when to finish meditating. If you still find it hard to clear your mind, you might try listening to an app or guided meditations which can be found online.

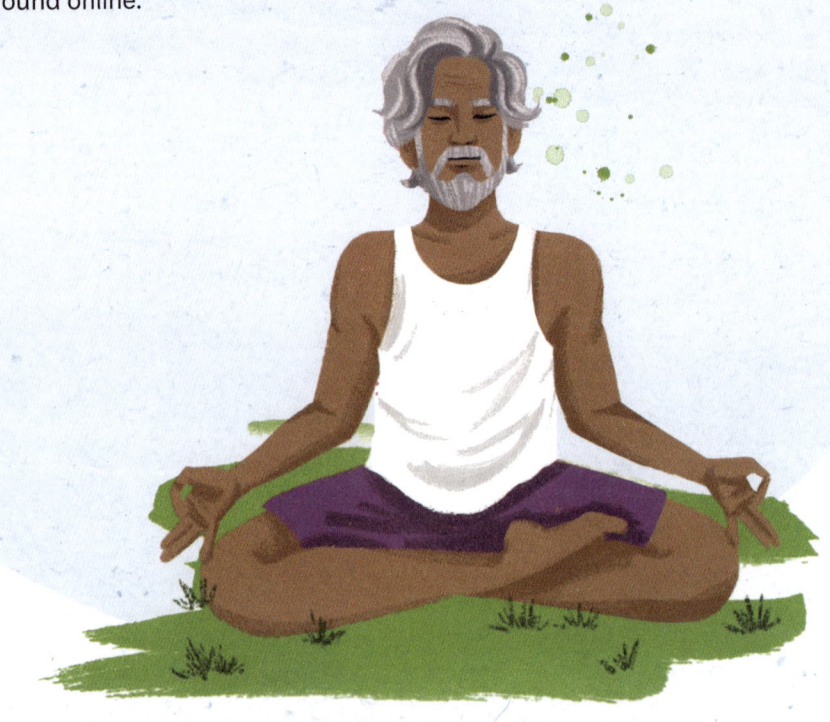

caring for your body

As explained in the chapter introduction, our appearance reflects the state of our body, and there are certain pillars of well-being we can address to improve our health and, in turn, how we look.

food and diet

We are what we eat. Food is fuel. Your body is a temple. These are just some approaches to eating, which, while simple, are generally true. A television advertisement I saw years ago showed a stomach having all sorts of alcohol, peanuts, and potato chips thrown into it, topped off by a heavy meal and another pint of beer! It was a great example of how not to eat. It is not that we should never eat junk food, but if we think before we start eating, we might not consume quite so much of it. Most things are okay in moderation, so if you smoke, drink alcohol or coffee, and eat sugary or junk foods, do so in moderation, remembering to respect your body and treat it kindly. If you wouldn't give it to your "child" self, think twice about giving it to your adult self.

Food combining is a method that is followed by some Buddhist monasteries, as well as a popular diet plan. The principle is to avoid eating carbohydrates and protein at the same meal, leaving a gap of around four hours between carbohydrates and protein. It allows the food you eat to travel through your system quickly, so you always feel light and energetic, and is a useful tool that can help with energy and weight control.

Food combining is an interesting concept that you might want to try, but is by no means the only way to eat healthily. There are myriad ways to eat, depending on culture, country of abode, taste, religion, and many other contributory factors, but so long as you eat predominantly fresh, wholesome food, and eat slowly and mindfully, you cannot go far wrong.

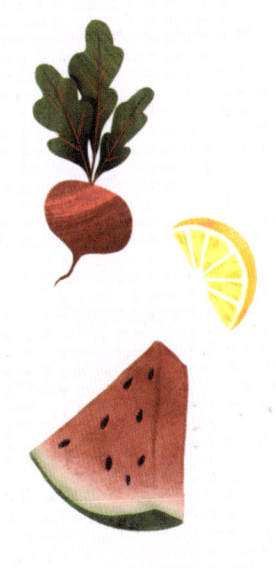

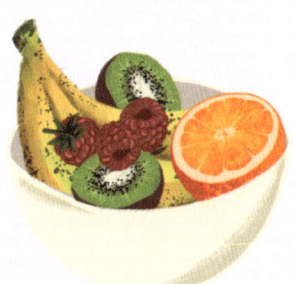

sleep

There is no disputing that a good night's sleep of 7–8 hours is optimal, but the reality is that not many people achieve it. Work, children, lifestyle, health, environment, and many other factors have an impact on how much or how little sleep we can get. Lack of sleep can have a really negative impact on our health, from lowering our immunity to turning us into stressful, sickly human beings. Even if your current situation doesn't allow for enough hours of sleep, here are a few tips to make sure the sleep you do have is of good quality.

- Make strategies that allow you to have a less cluttered mind when you go to bed—such as not watching action-packed or stressful material on the TV, checking your emails, or going to bed on an argument. Meditation can also help (see page 116).
- It is not good to eat just before you sleep, but if you have to and you are genuinely hungry, have a banana. The tryptophan, magnesium, and potassium in it will help you slumber.
- Don't drink too much water or tea before bed, to avoid needing to go to the bathroom in the night.
- Have an evening bath with relaxing essential oils.
- Make sure your bedroom is cool and dark, as well as uncluttered. Avoid having loads of detritus under your bed.
- Put a couple of drops of lavender essential oil on a handkerchief and place it under your pillow or wipe it over your bedding.
- Do the hand-breathing exercise from page 112 once you are in bed.
- Take a moment to think gratefully about your life, even if things aren't as perfect as you hoped—there is always something to be thankful for.
- Similarly, if children wake you up regularly, try not to be angry or stressed—instead, make them one of the things you are grateful for. It may be hard when you are sleep-deprived, but it is worth trying!

work

Your work will have an impact on your physical appearance. If you do something physical, your blood circulation should be in good shape, supporting your health and your glow. However, if you have a desk job, sitting down all day, make provision for some kind of movement in your day, whether it be walking to work, getting up and strolling around the office as much as possible without disturbing your work or others, drinking lots of water, going out in your lunch break, or even doing some seated exercises a couple of times during the day.

The facial yoga exercises for the eyes on pages 18–33 and the vagus nerve exercise on page 105 will help engage your parasympathetic nervous system (see page 102) and improve the way you feel if you are getting tired or stressed at work.

For overall wellness, it really helps if you enjoy your job, and that is certainly not a luxury everyone has. If this is the case for you, look for the positives in your work. Talk to coworkers and see how they feel, or take action to implement a change of job. Even just writing down what you wish you were doing could strike a chord in how to achieve it.

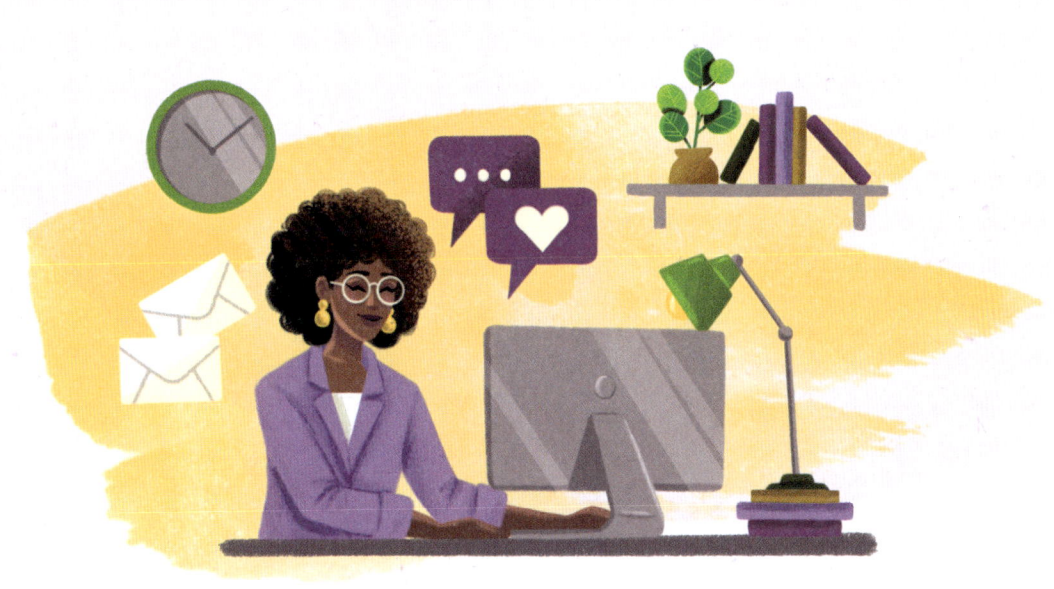

exercise

Exercise is vital for both your physical and mental health, but your ability, schedule, age, condition, and situation have an impact on how much you can do. However, with myriad ways to exercise, there is pretty much something for everyone.

Do more than one type of exercise per week if you can. Some types are good for stamina and strength, but yoga improves flexibility and focus, and Pilates increases core strength. Sports such as swimming and cycling have less impact than most and can be beneficial if you have an injury, but always check with a doctor or health professional first.

It is very important that you enjoy your exercise—it shouldn't be a chore. Never ask yourself whether you are feeling energetic enough for your chosen exercise class or session, because you will always feel great afterward.

Often, we don't even realize we are exercising. If running, working out at the gym, or doing karate or yoga are not for you, bear in mind that walking, housework, gardening, and playing with your children can all be a form of exercise, too. Walking, for example, can make an instant difference to how you are feeling. It can improve your mood, warm you up if you are cold, and give you a clearer head. It is never the wrong weather for it—simply wear the right clothes.

Exercising can be solitary or social. If you prefer having time to yourself, swimming, running, or cycling might be ideal options. Group or team sports are social, which can benefit your mental health—and your vagus nerve (see page 102).

Exercising outside will blow away the cobwebs and oxygenate your body brilliantly—a sure way of getting a natural glow. Plus, it offers an opportunity to top up your vitamin D! Yes, we must respect the dangers of too much sun and take the necessary precautions with hats and sunscreen, but do get out in the sunshine to soak up those happiness-making rays and that fresh air. Being outside is a blessing we should embrace.

dancing

Not only a form of exercise, dancing is fun, there is no doubt about it. It is such a natural thing to do that we don't think about all the benefits we get from it. Children naturally dance when they hear music from just a few months old. Their joy is contagious. Professional dancers put themselves through blood, sweat, and tears for the pure pleasure, freedom, and escapism dancing can offer. If you don't dance already, read these benefits of dancing for some sound reasons why you should put some music on and boogie in your kitchen:

- Boosts confidence
- Improves muscle tone
- Increases body strength and fitness
- Good for your heart, lungs, and circulation
- Gives you a better sense of balance and coordination
- Improves posture and flexibility
- Fires the limbic system (a part of the brain) to produce dopamine and serotonin, which make you happier and improve your mood
- Encourages social engagement (see page 105).

MAGICAL MELODIES

Music can instantly transport you to a better place. It can boost your energy or calm your nerves. Whether you are listening to music or playing an instrument, music has the power to change the way you feel. When you listen to something that reminds you of good times and joyous memories, it causes your brain to produce dopamine and serotonin, which are known to improve our mood and sense of well-being. Making music ourselves by singing or playing an instrument, whether we are a virtuoso or really bad at it, can put us in a state of "flow" or being "in the zone," which clears our minds of damaging thoughts.

caring for your body

mind and spirit

Nurturing our well-being is a holistic process—meaning that we must not only take care of our bodies, but also our minds. Everything is intertwined.

mindfulness

Mindfulness has grown in popularity in recent years and many people practice it. If you haven't heard of it, it is simply being mindful or aware of everything around you as much as possible, resulting in a calmer, happier, more considered you. It seems obvious that we should be more aware of people, our surroundings, our bodies, time, the weather, sound, food, fragrance, everything, but our natural state is to skim through life and take things for granted. Practicing mindfulness can improve every aspect of your life.

Jon Kabat-Zinn, founder of the Mindfulness Based Stress Reduction (MBSR) course, teaches nine pillars of mindfulness as a foundation for us to live by to create a more stress-free, happier life. These pillars are:

- Non-judging: It is not necessary to judge everything, though sometimes it seems like human nature. Try to rise above the temptation to judge when it is not necessary.
- Gratitude: There is so much to be grateful for. Give yourself time each day to list some of your blessings—on waking up and before you sleep are ideal moments to do this.
- Patience: Be patient with yourself and with others. Allow things to unfold.
- A beginner's mind: Be curious about all that is around you. Be open and receptive to everything you see.

- Trust: Trust in yourself and trust in others. Trust that everything will be alright. Anxiety never makes any outcome better.
- Non-striving: Of course, we all have to do our best, which could be construed as striving, but the essence of this tenet is to allow things just to flow. Be in the moment. Don't try to mend what is not broken.
- Acceptance: Things are not always as we want them to be. If we cannot or should not change something, we can accept it gracefully.
- Letting go: Non-attachment to thoughts or things allows our lives to flow more easily.
- Generosity: Giving to others, but also to yourself, simply for the joy and love it brings.

love

In *The Art of Letting Go*, the author David R. Hawkins says that every emotion has a vibration. This has been tested using kinesiology, a form of muscle testing that measures strength in the muscles when certain concepts or even items are introduced. It is useful to explore this concept as there is no doubt that when we are angry, sad, or afraid, we have little or no energy, and certainly no glow. All emotions have a physical and emotional effect on the body. When we are in love, we feel invincible, joyous, positive, and energetic. When we are angry, that too can give us energy but in the form of adrenaline, which, once spent, can leave us exhausted. Positive emotions are good for our health and well-being.

Hawkins' book does not expect you to leap from anger to love; rather, he suggests that you take small incremental steps to reach a feeling of love. This can be done by adopting an attitude of love for all things—a hard concept, but one to be considered. In fact, David Hawkins doesn't position love in first vibrational place—peace and joy are the front-runners. However, in daily life, the idea of love is a good place to start, and this will surely lead to joy and peace.

On the right, you'll find Hawkins' list of emotions in energetic vibrational order, peace being the highest and most aspirational emotion and shame the lowest and most energy-sapping. When you find your emotions reflecting any on this list, simply try to move your feelings to the next highest on the list and work your way up. You might not see a connection from one to the other at first. It is interesting, though, how when you actively think about it, the next emotion "up" is the one that will help you feel better.

The emotions:
- Peace
- Joy
- Love
- Reason
- Acceptance
- Willingness
- Neutrality
- Courage
- Anger
- Desire
- Fear
- Grief
- Apathy
- Guilt
- Shame

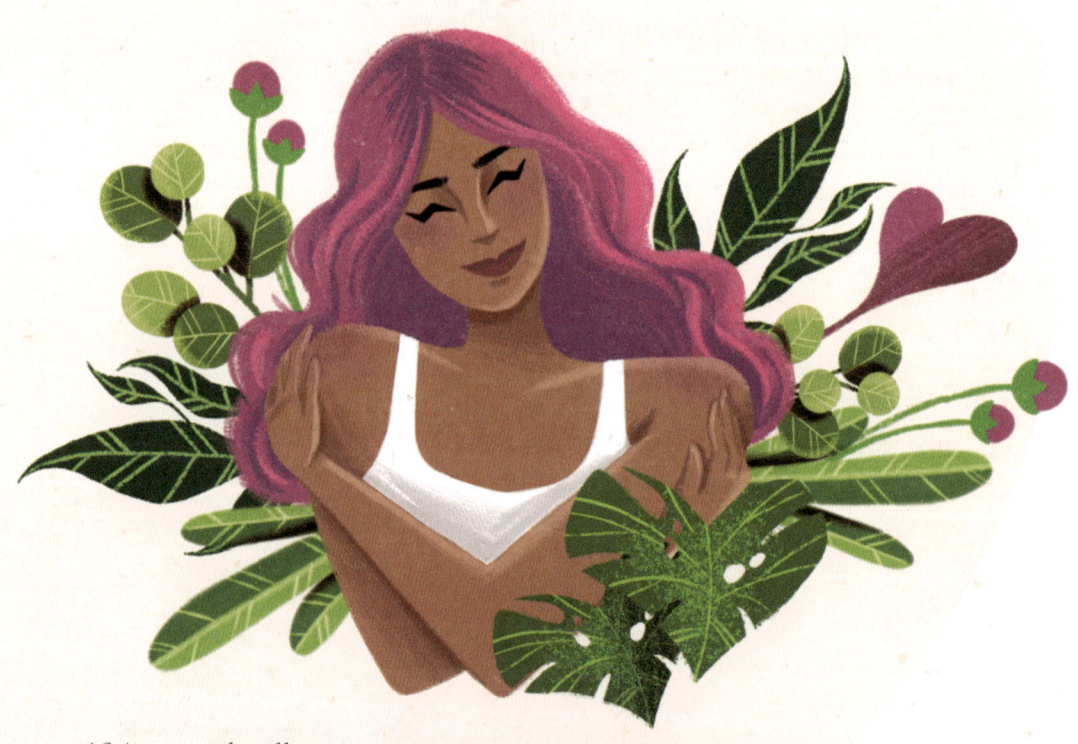

124   natural wellness

resources

Below are suppliers of natural products and tools you may need for facial yoga, reflexology, gua sha, and cryotherapy.

organic skincare products

For base oils and essential oils:

Angelico
www.angelico.london
Ships to UK only.

Balm Balm
balmbalm.com
Ships worldwide, except to EU.

Husk and Seed
huskandseedskincare.co.uk
Ships worldwide.

Inlight Beauty
inlightbeauty.co.uk
Ships and has stockists worldwide.

Naturally Balmy
www.naturallybalmy.co.uk
Ships to UK—contact regarding international delivery.

Neal's Yard Remedies
us.nealsyardremedies.com (US)
nealsyardremedies.com (UK)

Neve's Bees
nevesbees.co.uk
Ships to UK—contact regarding international delivery.

NHR Organic Essential Oils
nhrorganicoils.com
Ships worldwide.

UpCircle
us.upcirclebeauty.com (US)
upcirclebeauty.com (UK)
eu.upcirclebeauty.com (EU)

gua sha and cryotherapy tools

Natural Gua Sha
naturalguasha.com
Ships to US, Canada, UK, and Australia.

Pfefe
pfefe.com
Ships worldwide.

index

A
absolutes 95
acne face mapping 52
acupuncture 36, 104
alternate nostril breathing 114
antioxidants 82, 88
argan oil 81
around the clock 31
Ayurvedic medicine 52

B
balancing facial oil 96
base oils 78–83
bergamot 88
beta-carotene 79, 82
bloating 37
borage oil 83
box breath 113
breath push 33
breathwork 16, 110–16

C
calendula oil 81
cedarwood 91
chakras 39, 106–7
chamomile 87
cheeks, facial yoga 18, 26–7
chemicals in skin products 74
chi 36
circles (reflexology) 43
coconut oil 79
coherent breathing 112
cold water therapy 108–9
collagen 28, 59, 80, 82
connecting the dots 104
contact dermatitis 55
cooling breath 113
cranial nerves 102, 105
crow's feet minimizer 30
cryotherapy
   basic overview 59
   routine 70–1
   tools 61–2
   when to use 67

D
dancing 121
dermatitis 55
diet 117
dopamine 121

E
ear covering 44
effleurage 42
elastin 82
emotions
   facial mapping 54–5
   well-being 123–4
energizing breath 115
essential oils 76, 84–91, 94–5
exercise 14, 120
exfoliation 99
expression, changing 12
extended breath 115
eyes, facial yoga 19, 30–1

F
face, muscles 14
fascia 59
fish hooks 26
fish mouth 26
flavonoids 81, 88
flower waters 92
food 117
forehead
   facial reflexology 37
   facial yoga 20, 24–5
frankincense 91
frown-line reducer 24

G
GLA (gamma-linolenic acid) 83
grapefruit 88
gua sha
   basic overview 58–9
   benefits 59
   cautions 66
   method 64–7
   routine 68–9
   tools 60, 61
gut health 103

H
hand breath 112
horizontal-line reducer 25
hydrosols 75, 92–3
hydrotherapy 108–9

I
I Ching 38
infusions 80
intestines 102–4

J
jojoba oil 82

K
kiss kiss 28
kiss the sky 23

L
lavender 85
lemon essential oil 86
LI-20 104
lid and brow lift 31
limonene 88
linoleic acid 81
lip line reducer 29
love 123–4
lycopene 82
lymph 59, 66

M
macerations 80
mandarin 89
massage
   facial reflexology 46–7
   facial yoga 17
   LI-20 104
meditation
   breathwork 116
   chakras 106–7
meridians 36, 39, 40

mien shang 52–5
mind–body integration 53–5
mindfulness 122–3
mineral oils 76
mood
    serotonin 103, 121
    smiling 13
mouth
    facial reflexology 37
    facial yoga 21, 28–9
muscles
    face 14
    neck 14
music 121

N
nasal breathing 111
neck
    facial yoga 19, 22–3
    muscles 14
nervous system 102, 110
neurotransmitters 102
nighttime nourishing facial oil 97
nose
    facial reflexology 37
    facial yoga 21, 32–3

O
oils
    base oils 78–83
    basic overview 76
    essential oils 76, 84–91
    quality 95
    recipes 96–7
    storage 94–5
omega-6 fatty acids 81, 83

P
parasympathetic nervous system 102, 110
peach kernel oil 79
phytochemicals 88
pinching (reflexology) 43
plant oils 76
posture, yoga 16
pressing and moving (reflexology) 43
pressing (reflexology) 43

Q
qi 36, 52

R
raindrop fingers 17, 42
reflexology
    basic overview 36
    evening routine 48–51
    facial chakras 38–9
    facial mapping 52–5
    facial reflex zones 40–4
    forehead 37
    history 36–7
    mouth 37
    nose 37
    techniques 42
    tools 45
    warm up 46–7
relaxation
    facial reflexology 37
    facial yoga 15
resins 95
revitalizing morning facial oil 96
rose geranium 87
rosehip oil 82
routines
    cryotherapy 70–1
    facial yoga 18–21
    gua sha 68–9
    reflexology 48–51

S
sandalwood 90
scar reduction 59, 80, 88, 91
sebaceous glands 82
sensitive skin facial oil 97
serotonin 103, 121
serums 97
sleep 118
smiling
    benefits 12–13
    facial yoga 26
smoke lines 28, 29
social engagement 105
speech problems, facial yoga benefits 12
spine relaxation 37
starflower 83

steam 99
sunflower oil 80–1
supple neck 22

T
tapping 42
tea tree 86
Third Eye 24
tongue twister 28
Traditional Chinese Medicine (TCM) 36, 52, 104

V
vagus nerve 66, 102–5
vitamin A 79, 81, 82
vitamin E 79, 80, 81
vitamin E oil 80
vowel shape 22

W
walking 120
walking movement (reflexology) 44
warts 86
waterless skincare 74–5
work and wellness 119

Y
yoga
    basic overview 10
    benefits 11
    cheeks 18, 26–7
    developing routines 15
    eyes 19, 30–1
    forehead 20, 24–5
    massage 17
    meaning of word 10
    morning routine 18–21
    mouth 21, 28–9
    neck 19, 22–3
    nose 21, 32–3
    preparation 16–17

acknowledgments

Thank you so much to all these people:

CICO Books, for giving me the opportunity to share some of the knowledge I have gathered over the years.

My editor, Carmel Edmonds, who managed to pick up all my words like stitches on a knitting needle and put them in order. I truly believe you have a superpower, Carmel, and I have loved working with you.

Art director Sally Powell, designer Geoff Borin, and illustrator Camila Gray, for bringing my ideas and cell phone snapshots to life.

My daughter Megan and her husband Liam, for being models for those snapshots. It was really fascinating seeing them come to life as totally different people, nationalities, and ages.

My husband Haydn, for saving many bits of the book that I almost lost in the ether and for always encouraging me in whatever I do.

All my teachers over the years, especially my yoga teacher Debs, who will recognize her voice in parts of this book.

This has been fun!

photography credits

© CICO Books:
Pages 62–63: Roy Palmer.

© AdobeStock and the listed creators:

Page 1: ColorValley
Page 11: insta_photos
Page 28: Baan3d
Page 45: Pixel-Shot
Page 67: Lightfield Studios
Page 77: daffodfilred
Page 79: Mikhailov Studio
Page 90: Manon
Page 91: Olga Miraniuk
Page 94: TamiArita
Page 98: Syda Productions
Page 114: Bodil